Carl Jung
and Soul Psychology

Carl Jung and Soul Psychology

Karen Gibson
Donald Lathrop
E. Mark Stern
Editors

Harrington Park Press
New York • London • Sydney

ISBN 1-56023-001-0

Originally published as *VOICES: The Art and Science of Psychotherapy.* © 1986 by the American Academy of Psychotherapists. All rights reserved.

The Harrington Park Press edition is reproduced with the permission of the American Academy of Psychotherapists.

Harrington Park Press, 10 Alice Street, Binghamton, NY 13904-1580
EUROSPAN/Harrington, 3 Henrietta Street, London WC2E 8LU England
ASTAM/Harrington, 162-168 Parramatta Road, Stanmore (Sydney), N.S.W. 2048 Australia

Harrington Park Press is a subsidiary of The Haworth Press, Inc., 10 Alice Street, Binghamton, NY 13904-1580.

Library of Congress Cataloging-in-Publication Data

Voices, the art and science of psychotherapy.
    Carl Jung and soul psychology.

Originally published: Voices, the art and science of psychotherapy. American Academy of Psychotherapists.
    Bibliography: p.
    ISBN 1-56023-001-0
    1. Psychoanalysis. 2. Psychotherapy. 3. Jung, C. G. (Carl Gustav), 1875-1961. I. Stern, E. Mark, 1929-
BF173.J776V65   1986
150.19'54
1-56023-001-0   86-29497
                                                                    CIP

CONTENTS

E. Mark Stern
Editor of VOICES

Foundations for A Soul Psychology

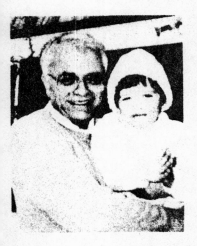

E. Mark Stern, Ed.D., completed his clinical studies at Columbia University (1955) and at the Institute of the National Psychological Association for Psychoanalysis. Besides his private practice in psychotherapy and psychoanalysis, Dr. Stern is Professor in the Graduate Division of Pastoral Counseling, Iona College, New Rochelle, New York, and is on the faculty of the American Institute for Psychotherapy and Psychoanalysis in New York City. Dr. Stern is a Diplomate in Clinical Psychology of the American Board of Professional Psychology and Fellow of the American Psychological Association.

215 East Eleventh Street
New York, New York 10003

Our Science is from the watching of shadows.

EZRA POUND
Canto LXXXV

Soul and Self

The soul in psychology? How best to claim a basis for its expression? Is there a prescribed design: one equipped to tap into sources of transcendence? And do these sources lead into possibilities for truth and good (Wojtyla, 1979)?

Hovering at the core of these enigmas is the challenge to exercise a self/awareness of soul. This exercise arouses the "contemplative emotions" (after Aquinas) and sanctifies awe, wonder, and surprise—all emotions which orient the self toward meaning.

The tacit awareness of the self rises out of personal integration and through reworking the disorganized pursuits of life into dynamic unity. Such unity indicates a significant relationship of self and soul. Self, now moving into an intimacy with meaning, draws attention to the multifaceted capacities of soul. And it is soul that ultimately sanctifies the boundless potential for developing personhood.

Soul as Unity

In its Platonic notion, *psyche* (soul), as well as its Hebrew equivalent *nephesh,* represents "the transhistoric depth of history" (Marcel, 1960, p. 269). Symbolized by a light within the darkness, soul is sometimes experienced as illuminative consciousness. As seen in the portrayal of saints, halos emphasize soulful qualities of transcendence. The aureole which appears to hover above the representations of saints redefines their transcendent boundaries. It's as if the halo unites the holy figure to that which is universal and etheric.

The etheric sensibilities are often characterized by birds in flight. Yet even here there is an interweaving correspondence between the nature of matter and spirit. In the biblical creation account, the aqueous turbulence is girdled by a crust of "firmament" (Genesis 1:6). Eventually, the spirit of creation is envisaged as a dove. In the romantic vision of William Blake, the firmament becomes the hazy circumference of the created universe, above and below which the soul quests on its dove-like journey to a spiritual reality (Frye, 1947).

In contemporary times quantum physics continues to relate and correlate wave (aqueousness/spirit) and particle (material creation). And while each is portrayed as homologous to the other, wave is, like the dove, often characterized as transcending particle. In this same sense, soul, although contiguous with the whole person, does conjure up a vision of transcendence. Wave/light/halo are figurative representations of soul, though they are coterminous with body/particle and with them form the complete person. In Freudian theory, the unconscious has the potential of representing itself consciously. This developmental sequence suggests the possibility of individuating (consciousness) the universal (unconscious). This realization of psychological unity, according to Andras Angyal (1941), ultimately involves "ethical and aesthetic attitudes as well as numerous forms of everyday behavior [that] seem to transcend the scope of a strictly individualistic life, and [anticipate] a definite trend toward superindividual goals" (p. 170).

As a dynamic Gestalt, such unity leads to an appreciation of the transcended superindividual whole even as its seemingly disparate elements form the hallmark of a workable order (Smuts, 1961). True unity is, however, never merely a collective sum of scattered parts. Soul is transcendent and as such exists as an expression of personal and collective wholeness. In these terms the so-called soul of a nation suggests an indefinable unity. For the individual, such unity provides an expanded sense of existence—one attained by what St. Thomas Aquinas might have termed an absolute unknowingness of the absolute known. In this spirit of the vital Gestalt, unity takes on a life of its own, erpressed and animated by the soul's mystery.

Soul as Vantage Point

The late mathematician/philosopher Alfred North Whitehead (1929) noted that a single mind contains the stunning capability of entering the

3

core of creation. Mind is that repeating event that "mirrors within itself the modes of the predecessors, as memories which are fused into its own content . . . [as well as having] a future [that] mirrors within itself such aspects [of that] . . . future [as are thrown] back on to the present" (p. 91). For Whitehead, newly excited by Einstein's relativity theory, the single moment stands as "subjective immediacy" unifying all disparity.

Carl Jung, through his own observations, commented on the mystery of unifying self or soul in the inspirational art form known as the "mandala." As an enduring Tibetan art form, the mandala depicts the Buddha, or local saint with Buddha nature, inside of a circle, yet separated into multiples of four, each multiple in its own circle portraying significant compassionate events in the life of the Buddha figure. A square, either contained in the circle or surrounded by it, indicates the embracing unity of the circle. In Jungian thinking, mandala moves beyond transcendental idealism and through it to the realization of soul. Here soul is ultimate Gestalt as it gradually surfaces as unity of individual ego and universal compassion.

Related to the mandala experience is William James' (1890/1950) use of the term, "stream." Stream confirms the processive unity of self/ soul and creation/superindividuality. James himself "confessed" that while there might well be a "rigorous answer to [the] question of the soul's continuity" or "its relation to . . . other objects," it is "in the present world [that] minds precede, succeed, and coexist with each other in the common receptacle of time, and in their collective relations" (pp. 199-200).

In practice soul transcends ego even as it mobilizes self. Beyond fear and apprehension of ego, soul remains the self's mode of expansion. As the primary means of transcending ego, soul highlights creativity and encourages superindividual engagement.

Despite its collective intention, soul personalizes, even as it integrates the whole universe. Nevertheless, soul is integrative only as it provides expanded opportunities for individual *choice*. It is only through personal preference that the individual is able to respond to the superindividual. Soul provides a vehicle for achieving personal integration as it equates with communal wholeness. According to psychologist-theologian Victor White (1952), cognition, in its sacred covenant with soul, breaks "the shell of [the] small 'I' . . . [and] forges an existential link . . . with God and the cosmos" (p. 249). Soul psychology exists to understand this covenant.

Soul Psychology

Soul psychology seeks, among other things, to notate what the individual experiences as ontological insecurity. It considers moments of anxious insecurity as opportunities for the appreciation of unified fields.

Such fields have been posited as providing soul with "real meetings with other realities" (Buber, 1957, p. 82). This participation with the mystery of the Whole unites seemingly disparate experiences. In the light of soul psychology personal history—the past, present, future—is united. Past is thus redeemed and emancipated by the present. According to a common French truism, *on ne guérit pas on se souvenant, mais on se souvient en guérissant* (one does not heal by remembering but one remembers as the outcome of healing). Each life event in its own time is radically responsive to the timelessness of universal unconscious. Unity is thus recognized despite ambivalence. What has been referred to as ambivalence is, according to soul psychology, nothing more than partial vision or the ambiguous Gestalt and as such constitutes the possibility of divinity.

Carl Jung (1971, 1975) must be credited with the vision of a psychic totality capable of bridging ambivalence. To Jung (1975) the heartland of the psyche remains "divinely created nature" (p. 237), challenging the self to engage the fullness of creation. For Jung, only as ego gives way can self expand and begin to know "that inasmuch as one is oneself one is also the other" (p. 237). Segments of Jung's correspondence focus on the self's relationships to the broader collective unconscious. "Individuation," for Jung, is "the process of becoming whole and holy." To Victor White he writes of "the oneness of the self [containing a] divine spark within its inviolable precincts" (p. 242).

For Jung (1977), individuation, in order to be authentic, must ultimately extend to the universal. In Jungian terms, the ancestral soul reaches into the collective of humankind while the personal soul develops an awareness of its individual mission. By way of archetypes, individuation implies a steady incremental awareness of the superindividual.

Archetypes are particularized inclinations of an emerging universal consciousness. An appreciation of the archetypes remains foundational to individuation inasmuch as they serve both individually and collectively as bridges to soul.

Archetypes as Elements of Balance

John Weir Perry (1970), a Jungian analyst and psychiatrist, found that two or more archetypes often blend together as syndromes-struggles in persons wrestling with the outer bounds of sanity. In this sense archetypes emerge as opportunities for bringing order to balancing opposites. Borderline and/or schizophrenic experiences are often sensitive to the workings of archetypes since they are representations of a collective creative engagement. For the recovering schizophrenic, struggling with a tenacious surreal view of life, the realization of archetypes often serves as opportunity for confronting and assimilating a sense of universal

5

balance. According to Perry, assimilation of one or more archetypes in the schizophrenic may awaken some key healing experiences, such as:

Location at a world center;

death and afterlife;

a return to the beginning of time;

a cosmic conflict or battle;

a threat from the opposite [sex] (Here I think of the embattlement of anima struggling with the animus and vice versa);

a sacred marriage (Perhaps an integration of anima and animus);

a new birth or rebirth; and

a new society.

As nonlinear developmental phases, archetypic blendings appear to act as an ensemble of forces contributing to the workings of the soul.

The Soul's Task

Certainly there can be no hidebound picture of personal development. Nonetheless, the integration of archetypes suggests unity and confluence. Taking a lead from Perry's schema, no one, sane or insane, can be spared the obligation of transcending fragmentation. The unifying task reaches into the deepest recesses of self. Authentic well-being is thus based on intimations of a universal ground of all being. Once only seen in shadow, the archetypes eventually unite in the workings of the soul. The unification of these archetypes remains both the mystery as well as the realization of transcendence and love.

Within the context of soul psychology, each personal struggle anticipates an assent to the purpose of existence. As a true psychology of transcendence, the content of soul psychology ultimately underlies all other polemics and dialectics. And as psychotherapy, soul psychology fosters what Rollo May (1969) has termed the "communion of consciousness" through which and in which "love and will . . . are both present in each genuine act . . . [so that] we mold ourselves and our world simultaneously" (p. 325).

* * *

The essays in this volume seek to expound on the identity and unifying work of soul psychology. Psychotherapy is profoundly indebted to Carl Jung, who among others, discovered the mappings of soul psychology. Doctors Donald Lathrop and Karen Gibson have met a monumental challenge in enlisting the scope of wisdom you are about to encounter in these pages. The dedication of Doctors Gibson and Lathrop provides us with a solid basis for an understanding of the foundations of soul psychology.

REFERENCES

Angyal, A. (1941). *Foundations for a science of personality.* New York: Commonwealth Fund.

Buber, M. (1957). *Eclipse of God: Studies in the relation between religion and philosophy.* New York: Harper Torchbooks.

Frye, C. (1947). *Fearful symmetry: A study of William Blake.* Princeton: Princeton University Press.

James, W. (1950). *Principles of psychology* (Authorized Edition). New York: Dover Publications. (Original work published 1890).

Jung, C. (1952). Forward. In V. White, *God and the unconscious.* London: Havill Press.

Jung, C. (1971). *Psychological types. The psychology of individuation* (H. G. Baynes, Trans.). New York: Harcourt Brace.

Jung, C. (1975). *Letters* (G. Adler & A. Jaffe, Eds.; R. F. C. Wuld, Trans.), (Vol. 2). Princeton: Princeton University Press.

Jung, C. G. (1977). *Jung speaking: Interviews and encounters* (E. McGuire & R. F. C. Hull, Eds.). Princeton: Princeton University Press.

Marcel, G. (1960). *The mystery of being.* Chicago: Gateway Edition.

May, R. (1969). *Love and will.* New York: Norton.

Perry, J. W. (1970). Jung and analytical psychology. In C. P. Rosenbaum, *The meaning of madness: Symptomatology, sociology, biology and therapy of the schizophrenias,* (pp. 250-258). New York: Science House.

Smuts, J. C. (1961). *Holism and evolution.* New York: Macmillan.

Whitehead, A. N. (1929). *Process and reality.* London: Cambridge University Press.

Wojtyla, K. (1979). The person: Subject and community. *The Review of Metaphysics, 33*(130), 273-308.

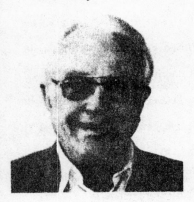

Donald Lathrop
Consulting Editor for this issue

Psychotherapy and Soul

My soul's journey is largely in the underworld. Dante's *Inferno* is my favorite travelogue. My daily work as a psychotherapist is an essential part of my own individuation process. That is one of the times when I feel most whole, most complete. Other activities that lead to the same feeling are writing, making love, and cutting wood. My essential self-therapy tools are dreamwork and keeping a journal.

111 West Curling
Boise, Idaho 83702

Soul psychotherapy is the applied science of soul psychology. Soul psychology is the science of the soul. What is soul?

However we currently define it, soul is back in the language of everydayness. No less enduring a literary journal of Americana than *Esquire* magazine devoted its June 1985 issue to the subject "The Soul of America" subtitled, "Two years ago, *Esquire* went looking for the real America; we found it." That is in bold print on the cover; there is no female body to grab the eye of the newsstand shopper, just large black print on a white background. Lee Eisenberg's (1985) opening statement describes their editorial process, which was suitably feminine (that is, indirect, intuitive, self-evolving). The trueness of their collective, Manhattan, high-rise, slick-magazine-publisher brainstorming is revealed by their conclusions:

> A breakthrough came when we realized that we hadn't been talking about the difference among regions so much as *the very essence* of the *American identity*. That is, if there is such a thing as the American character, its soul lies in *the sum total of values* that exist distinctly in a multitude of places. (p. 17) (Italics mine)

Soul is essence, the sum total of values. It is that quality which is quintessential for the whole. It is not quantitative. It has no geographical location. It is not limited to living entities nor to objects having material substance. (For example, a group—which is solely a mental construct and has no objective existence—may have a soul.) Soul is a quality, not a property. Soul is a vibration of the bundle of light of which all matter consists. Soul is perceptible only by psyche. Soul alone perceives itself. It is soul in us which interacts with soul in things, in situations, in experiences.

Psychology is the science of the psyche. Soul psychology is one tiny part of the whole, but its subject (soul) is the essence of the psyche. Soul psychology is the study of the essence of the psyche, of the roots and origins of *all* of our values, the dark as well as the light, lunar as well as solar. The soul's journey is revealed in dreams and in deeds. It is the paradox between what we believe ourselves to be (ego consciousness's self-concept) and what we are in our essence that engages the soul psychotherapist.

Soul psychology is depth psychology. Freud opened the door to the scientific study of the soul. Sexuality is the language of the soul. Jung took the next step, which was to penetrate the transpersonal realm of soul, the deepest layers of psyche where we merge with body and the material universe on one end and with spirit and the non-material on the other end of the spectrum.

Soul is the creator. Soul psychology studies the creative process. It is a modern outgrowth of alchemy, of the pre-science which plumbed the depths in search of the secret of creation. Soul psychology, like alchemy, is a phenomenological method—one observes and describes what is. One describes without presuming to explain. The master remains aware that what is observed and what observes are one, that it is through soul that we perceive and relate to soul.

Soul psychology describes the effects of "invisible," non-material forces on observable phenomena, all of which are ultimately the psyche of the observer. Psyche is both observed and observes in all encounters with soul. There is no possibility of "objective" (i.e., an external relationship between soul and psyche) observation, description, or measurement.

This fact, of soul being a necessary "contaminant" of all studies of soul, is the cause of all of the confusion, conflict, and contention about the nature of soul. It was the alchemist who initiated the scientific study of soul. We, like Jung, are the beneficiaries (perhaps even the results) of those pioneering experiments into the very nature of essence. As our science has become ever more literal, as our consciousness has become ever more concretized and materialistic, the search for soul has become more and more imperative.

Soul psychotherapy is an applied science of soul psychology. Psychotherapy is the laboratory of the soul psychologist. All soul psychologists are inevitably psychotherapists. Each treatment relationship is an experiment in which "the method" is employed in the attempted transmutation of the base material of disease to the pure gold of enlightened self-knowledge. It is in the experience of his or her own depth therapy/ analysis that the novice begins initiation. As was true of the alchemical pre-figuration of soul psychology, countless students try to learn "the method" by cookbook approaches. These counterfeit pseudo-adepts reflect one of the basic soul disorders of Americans—the belief in the short-cut, the quick fix, effortless transformation.

I was initiated into soul psychotherapy by psychotic women on the wards of New Orleans' Charity Hospital where I began my studies in psychiatry. Many other soul psychotherapists have been led to this secret cult by recognizing their schizophrenic patients as teachers, *par excellence,* of depth psychology. Jung was one such person. He listened respectfully to the lunatic ravings of his patients at Burgholzi. In time, he discovered the basic structural elements of the psyche, the archetypes (archaic + typical), for those experiences.

It was while working with the chronic psychotics that Jung began his word-association experiments. He noticed that people had delayed response times as well as idiosyncratic responses to certain words in the standard word-association-test list he was presenting. He inferred that these specific words had stimulated an emotionally laden cluster of thoughts, feelings, images in that individual. He named these clusters *complexes.* Later, he identified the core around which the complex had accumulated as the archetype. Both the complex and its archetypal core can be labeled by examining the stimulus word, the response words, and the subject's associations and memories brought into consciousness by the stimulus word. Thus, if *anger* elicits *fear* or *hurt* or *towering* and if these lead to *father* in that individual, we would recognize this as the father complex and its core as the father archetype. Likewise, we find the mother, brother, sister, god, goddess, ego, soul, and so on. There is no comprehensive list of the archetypes, nor can there be.

I find it helpful to imagine the archetypes as being analogous to the genes—the protein molecues that make up the 96 human chromosomes. The genes are finite but the possible combination of genes is infinite. So are the possible combinations of archetypes and complexes. Archetypes are the "genes" of the psyche. They are the templates upon which the individual form of the complex is built. Like genes, archetypes reveal themselves by their effects. Unlike genes, they can never be "seen" directly. Archetypes manifest as images, in dreams, in fantasy, in creative expression. They manifest as personality types and traits, as neurotic symptoms, as physical illness, as personal myths (life-script), as every aspect of existence.

Psychological constructs, such as archetypes, complexes, self, object relations, and others, are the essential tools of the psychotherapist. They are the retorts, the containers, for our alchemical experiments. But laboratory equipment does not make a scientist and concepts do not make a therapist, a healer. Just hanging around crazy people, even living with them as some pioneers of soul psychotherapy did, does not transform a psychologist into a healer. There remains the issue of the therapist's own soul and of its "redemption." The crucible for that redemption is personal therapeutic analysis. I'm not referring to those sterilized de-souled euphemisms of denial of one's own soul wound called "didactic" or "training" analysis. I am certainly not talking about weekend or week-long or month-long or year-long or life-long experiential groups. No shaman ever emerged from sitting around the campfire swapping clinical tidbits with the other acolytes. Personal therapy of the therapist is the beginning of the acknowledgment of the soul wound.

Soul psychotherapy is a contemporary shamanic form which has arisen out of the loss of soul in the industrialized, urbanized, literalized, materialized modern world. Psychology is the secular religion of this world. Television is the church. Soul psychology is a heretical, underground, anti-establishment movement. Soul psychotherapists are witches, warlocks, madmen and madwomen who have wrested something personal from their apprenticeships (credentialing programs and personal therapy).

In earlier forms of civilization, the shaman (male or female) was identified in childhood, sometimes at birth, often at the threshhold of adolescence. He or she was, is, *different,* deformed in some special way that sets him or her apart. Soul speaks through the wound, through our differentness, our deformity. In our society, depth analysis/therapy is one of the rituals of initiation into the shamanic path, the life that is ruled by soul. That our lives are dedicated to, directed by, soul merely makes us different, neither better nor worse. We do have a sacred trust, a responsibility, but so do the rest. For all of us, the ultimate commandment is "To thine own soul be true." There is not a day of clinical work that passes in which our trueness is not tested.

My own recognition of the true nature of my work as a psychotherapist came through via a characteristically mundane development. When I moved my family to California in 1970, my first marriage was in a black *nigredo* state. We moved from New Orleans, birthplace of America's soul music—jazz—to Los Angeles, birthplace of the soul-less images that carry America's dominant religion—movies, TV. Ego psychology and behaviorism, both soul-less systems, were ascendant. Fritz Perls and Eric Berne had given birth to Werner Erhard who had, in turn, taught people to know they were alive by experiencing the sensation of a full bladder!

In the midst of my personal journey and within this social retort, I found myself in a new land, a land of (among other things) personalized license plates. Of course, all the good ones had been taken—"SHRINK," "THERAPY," "PSYCH." There was no competition for the label that came to me as I struggled with who I was/am—"SOUL DR." I have been soul doctor ever since.

It is the soul that "does" the psychotherapy just as it is the soul that is "therapized." The life of the soul psychotherapist is directed by, lived by, if you will, his or her soul. There is an intimate, personal, love/hate relationship between the ego and the soul of the soul psychotherapist. This is not romantic love. This is the love that comes with knowing, with years of living together in the same body, of communicating through the same mind.

Is soul inherently "good" and thus the practitioner of the soul's medicine anointed by benevolence? Need I ask?

Evil has its soul and soul has its own morality, the morality of nature. Indeed, it is the dark side of the soul that occupies the psychotherapist. No one seeks help other than from concern with the dark side. Hades is the god of soul psychotherapy.

"How do you do, Peter. I'm Don Lathrop." I usher this 43-year-old, well-dressed, pleasant man into my living-room-style office. "Have a seat." He sits tentatively on the end of the long sofa opposite the wing-back chair I usually occupy. My consulting room is small, well lit by three large windows in the heavy stone walls of the corner of this turn-of-the-century building. It is decorated in warm earthtone colors accented by blue-grey trim. This place once served as quarters for the staff of the orphanage, the neighboring large stone building on Warm Springs Avenue which is now a children's treatment clinic.

"Tell me your situation, Peter. I don't know anything about you other than that you got my name out of the phone book and called to make an appointment." The man sitting opposite me fidgets momentarily, sits forward on the soft cushioned couch, clears his throat, looks straight at me and says, "I molested my daughter. I need help."

Did he catch that immediately inhibited blink of my eyes? Maybe he didn't, but his soul did. He's looking right at me, reading my instinctive response to his opening statement.

"Tell me about it." I take a quick sip from my coffee mug, arrange the manila folder and note paper on my lap. My pen is poised to write, to give me something to do while this stranger and I decide whether to let each other into our lives.

Fear, revulsion, disgust, self-pity, anger, uncertainty sweep over me as Peter tells his story. It's a familiar story to me; but it is *his* story, *his* suffering, to him. There is no way I can protect myself from feeling this man's pain by putting his words through the "clinical" part of my mind. Psychological concepts help me to contain my own anxiety, my own pain, my own awakened complexes.

"I don't know why I did it. I knew it was wrong! I told myself I was 'teaching' her, that I was showing her how to enjoy her body." No need to comment. This man has already faced his own superficial rationalizations. He is afraid. He knows the power of those forces within that thrash the ego about when it has fallen victim to its own sense of being all there is, of being in charge of the psyche.

"She was nine when I started. Her mother and I were not getting along. We were fighting a lot. I used to spend a lot of nights on the couch in the living room. One night I went in and lay down with my little girl. I needed someone to hold me. I needed to be close to someone. I needed someone to touch me—to touch my private parts, you know. . . ."

"You put your little girl's hand on your cock?"

"Yeah, that's what I mean." He pauses, a bit flustered.

Profanity, vulgarity—"gutter language," my mother called it—that is part of the vocabulary of the soul. These feelingful, emotionally charged words and expressions connect with a baser, more primal part of us. The more urgent my need to make contact, the more intense the moment in the therapeutic relationship, the more I use the language despised by the educated, cultured, polite.

My first job after I moved to California in 1970 was as ward psychiatrist for one of the acute psychiatric wards at Los Angeles County Hospital. I ran my ward as a therapeutic community—as well as I could in that monolithic public hospital. First thing each day we gathered everyone together in the day room, about 40 staff and patients. The only people excused were those so assaultative they had to be kept in locked seclusion. The crazed folks off the streets of America's crucible—suicidal, psychotic, homeless, acutely and chronically mentally ill—met for the first time with their psychiatrist, nurses, technicians, ward clerk, and with patients who had been on the ward for one to 30 days. Urgency, intensity were the normal mood. I spoke in the language of the people, the language of the gutter, the language of the hospital. Nurses complained to the Director of Nurses. I was called down, questioned, counseled, warned. In the end, I was "let go" on the final day of my 6-month probationary period. It did not matter that there had not been a single suicide of my patients in 6 months, nor that our ward got people on their feet and able to function faster than any of the other wards. In the end, it was the pious and the righteous who had the last word. When he fired me, the director suggested that my methods might better be tried in the private sector where patients could choose not to be subjected to the "abuse" of confrontation, passion, and profanity. I have since had the privilege of practicing soul psychotherapy, profanity and all, in another therapeutic community in a public institution. The Boise V.A. inpatient psychiatric service became a powerful arena for the reclamation of men damaged in Vietnam as well as in the towns and cities of Idaho. While my style provoked great anxiety, the more personal climate in Boise made my acceptance quite the opposite of Los Angeles.

Sexuality is the primary arena of soul. The words and sounds we use to communicate sexually are full of primary energy. Sex is soul in action. "Making love," "fucking," "screwing," "getting it on," are each different experiences. None of them is copulation, which isn't even an experience; it is a concept.

Calling a cock a penis, or genitals, or private parts, does not stir the emotion-laden complex. Each of us has words that are keys to unlocking the emotion—cock, dick, pecker, prick, prong, pork, meat, schlong, pee-pee, weiner—the patient knows his or her own soul language. This must become part of the exchange in therapy if soul is to be involved.

This man sitting across from me in the safe haven of my consulting room knows that I am one of the keys to his keeping himself out of prison. Thousands of men like Peter will have their first exposure to psychological self-exploration as an alternative to prison, because of our societal response to child abuse.

The individual with severe soul sickness may have no subjective pain, no awareness of the severity of his or her condition. The person does experience fear, but the focus of the fear may be on externals—like going to prison—rather than on the awesome power and extremity of one's own dark side.

"I didn't mean to hurt her. I don't know why I did it. I tried to stop but I couldn't." He appeals to me with his voice, his eyes, his tensely clasped hands. He wants me to understand. He expects me to understand. I expect myself to understand.

Fools, we are both fools. I cannot give him absolution. I can listen. I can try to teach him to listen. I can care. With a lot of time and effort and much, much more pain that I dare admit to myself, I can perhaps help him to feel what his child felt—betrayed, used, manipulated, exploited—and still be able to love. Perhaps. And perhaps his daughter, now exploding into adolescence, will permit trust to seep back into her heart as my co-therapist/wife, Karen Gibson, leads her gently by the hand through her own soul-healing therapy. And perhaps all of us together, through the medium of family therapy, will be able to find the gold, the transformation, in this dark journey.

Aggression gone berserk is humanity's most compelling soul dilemma. Whether as cancer in our bodies, child abuse in our families, or nuclear arms deployment on our spaceships, the danger to soul is the same.

The soul of America (not the *Esquire* soul but that more elemental essence that reveals itself in our history) speaks to many moderns through

Native American wisdom. In that tradition, the ultimate test of the validity of all decisions of the tribal council is "No law shall be passed that will harm the children (meaning all life, not just human)." In the consulting room, in the living room, and in the legislature, this is still sound soul ecology.

REFERENCE

Eisenberg, L. (1985, June). Backstage with Esquire. *Esquire,* p. 17.

Karen Gibson

Consulting Editor for this issue

Soul Psychology:
A Native American and Jungian Dance

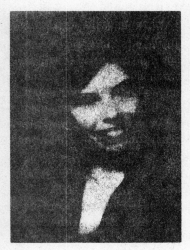

My soul's dance has led me through studies with Native American medicine people, Jungian analysis, and a doctoral dissertation on the reemergence of the feminine principle.

I am in private practice. My office is in my home, making my daily life and professional practice interrelated. My special interest is in the creation and use of ritual—in psychotherapy; in my family; and in my community, relating to 17 third-grade girls, one of whom is my daughter, Amy. This is both the most conventional and radical expression of my feminist being.

111 West Curling
Boise, Idaho 83702

Soul is difficult to speak of, more so to write about. Soul must be felt, experienced. Soul is not containable, controllable. Soul is the feminine principle in life. She is psychic energy with which we can dance. She has her own timing and will never be possessed by the ego. She can be related to or betrayed by woman or man. She has no sexual preference. She is not the province of woman or man. Soul is mysterious, deep, dark, unpredictable. She is life-giving and life-taking. She erupts spontaneously. She does not conform to our expectations. She is amoral. Sometimes, she is difficult to reach and may only communicate to us through our awareness of her absence. Soul is essence, the beginningless beginning. It is usually through our hearts that we feel our souls.

Spirit is the creative energy that moves the soul into manifestation. Spirit initiates. Spirit discriminates. Spirit is focus. Spirit orders and structures. Spirit is intent and intense. Spirit is the masculine principle, an essential life force in man and woman. He moves the personal into a larger context thereby deepening understanding and meaning. Through the mind we feel our spirit.

If the soul is not connected to the spirit, its expression may never get beyond the limits of the body. If the spirit is unconnected to the soul, its manifestation in the outer world is a glorification of the ego rather than a reflection of one's essence. Soul and spirit live within the body, our earth lodge. Matter is as sacred as soul and spirit.

A Navajo medicine woman once said to me, "Remember, you are the column through which the sun and the earth make love." Standing with an awareness of my feet solidly supported by the earth and my arms stretching up to the sky where the sun was directly oppositional to the earth at noon, I felt a union of body, soul, and spirit. Jungians terms this *coniunctio,* the bringing together of opposites. Native Americans call it *walking in balance.*

Cheyenne medicine man and author Hyemeyohst Storm (1972) envisions spirit as boundless energy, beautiful and perfect in all ways except one. Spirit has no understanding of limitation, no experience of substance. Spirit is total energy of the mind without body or heart. Spirit comes to the earth to learn the things of the heart through touching (p. 7).

Through our bodies we participate in the Great Mysteries—birth, growing, changing, aging, dying. In mid-life we begin to feel within ourselves what we have seen in nature: the birth, death, rebirth cycle. This may either be a time of deep psychological growth or a time when a person expends a lot of psychic energy in denial. Jung (1934/1960) clearly states that the goal of the second half of life is death. The Indians say it is time to make death your ally. Death is the Giveaway. In death one form gives up its material identity so that another form can live. The buffalo to Indian people is the symbol of the Giveaway. Through death the buffalo fed, clothed, and sheltered his people. The spirit of the buffalo chose death so that the people could live. Indian hunters understood they were recipients of a sacred gift not counting coup. The Sun Dance teaches that movement is change. Change is life. Change is death. Death becomes life through the Giveaway. Our psychological experience of growth follows the same process—the cyclical process of life. The ordinary is extraordinary.

The same process of linking spirit, soul, and matter can be experienced from the introverted attitude. An inner image or feeling awakens the soul. The person dances the image within until a readiness to manifest it is stirred. Then a poem is written or some other form of expression occurs. The creation may be artistic, intellectual, or relational. Regardless of its form there is movement into the material world and return to the inner world.

The religious experience occurs in those moments when the soul, spirit, and body spontaneously are one and the person is filled with awe, humility, knowing, and feeling. The effect of that moment continues long after the moment has died. There is a strong desire to tell someone of the experience, along with fear of being seen as crazy and irrational. The material itself, the essence of the experience, demands communication and manifestation. Mythos means communication. Myths are communications of spiritual experiences.

In answer to a question posed during a lecture on alchemy, Marie

Louise von Franz (1980), a student of Jung's and my favorite interpreter of him, emphasizes that the religious experience flows naturally into manifestation because it is real. She illustrates the necessity of communicating a religious experience through Black Elk's story. While in a coma at age nine, Black Elk had a powerful spiritual experience which he kept to himself until he developed a thunder phobia. He consulted a medicine man who told him his experience was not given to him only. He was instructed to tell his people. When he told the tribe of his visions, the thunder phobia disappeared (pp. 260-261).

The religious experience is both private and personal and part of the community. The personal experience links us to the archetypal, to a large context, to the tribe, that is, the collective.

My understanding of the interrelatedness of mind, body, and spirit; and of individual to community, personal to archetypal, is deepened as I explore Jungian psychology and Native American traditions. The marriage of these two perspectives was sparked by a common experience many women share—having a baby. It was the first time I experienced an amazing personal, physical experience and simultaneously felt possessed by the archetype. Giving birth was an experience of life beyond my control. My task was to work in cooperation with the process that began itself. As the magic of those moments faded into past memory, and the reentry into the complexities of ordinary day-to-day existence came into the foreground, I understood what I had formerly vehemently opposed in Don Juan's teachings to Castaneda regarding women having children. Don Juan said when a woman has a baby, that leaves a hole in her soul. I felt that hole. I needed to reclaim Karen. Surely it was true that I knew I couldn't mother Amy if I lost myself, but my motivating instinct was not so noble. I wanted all of me as woman to live, not just the mother. My task was to reclaim myself from the identification with, and possession by, the Great Mother. My post-partum depression was a loss of soul.

The place for me to start was the physical. I knew this intuitively and acted on it. I felt a need to reclaim my body which had been partially on loan for 9 months and still was through breast-feeding. I decided to start running. Down the hill from my home lived an elderly couple who were happy to care for Amy while I took time for myself. So I marked off a mile along the dusty road that followed the winding Snake River. A mile didn't seem very long until I tried to run it. The dry, hot August heat seemed to create an impenetrable space. I felt fear as I unsuccessfully repeated my ritual. Then one day as I was running, feeling defeated and depressed, an image of an Indian runner overtook me. Before I knew it I was past my mile marker. I stopped, turned around, and experienced what my Catholic upbringing had taught me to know as a moment of grace. To the Indian, it would be described as a moment when the earth stood still. I walked the mile back home feeling balanced while experiencing an intensification of awareness, both inner and outer, that felt magical indeed. Thereafter I took Amy for walks along the river. We would talk to the wind, the bugs, the water, the wildlife. In the native sense I was introducing Amy to all her relations. I had no idea how important this ritual was to me until a local newspaper reporter was doing a human-interest story on me and my husband as therapists raising their child. She asked about religious training. When my husband told her we had no plans in that area I described these walks, explaining their deep spiritual nature and pointing out a child's senses as her first avenue of learning. I felt something speaking through me very clearly, powerfully, and with emotion.

The Indian runner is a reflection of the man within, a positive animus figure, my spirit. He was a gift from my unconscious to heal my soul and to connect me to my body and to the material world. In days gone by, the Indian runner was a messenger. He scouted ahead of the tribe to bring back information necessary to facilitate movement into unknown territory. During the buffalo hunt, the runner's job was to find the buffalo, run amidst the herd, pacing the animals and leading them to the edge of the cliff where they would fall to their death. The runner's job and the buffalos' death were essential to the life of the people.

The Indian runner in my psyche connects my inner and outer worlds. He teaches me the value of paying attention to details in both worlds, a way of perceiving that is not natural to me. He leads me into new experiences with aloneness, teaching me the meaningfulness of relationships with things other than people. He reflects the power of the imaginal realm while connecting me more closely to the external material world. I am learning the value of not being seen or heard while experiencing a new way of seeing and hearing. I am learning to stalk as well as to dream. Through the Indian image, I feel more deeply connected to my feminine nature; I also have a deeper understanding and respect for interplay of the masculine/feminine, soul/spirit dynamics in my psyche and in the outer world.

I am neither an Indian by blood nor a Jungian by certification but my soul has been touched by both. I hear the same wisdom in both. The language and metaphors are different. Interlacing them into the fabric of my life and work is my current conscious focus. The process, however, was happening long before I knew it.

The human pull toward wholeness, the process Jung termed individuation, is what the Native Americans called the warrior's path with heart. "God" to the Indians was the presence of wholeness; to Jung the Self. God or the Self is not experienced directly. It is experienced symbolically, in dreams and visions, and, to the Indians, it is continually present in nature.

Jung's ideas about psychological types and the teachings of the medicine wheel both acknowledge that each human is born into this world with a medicine, a power, an innate pattern of ego adaptation that determines his or her habitual frame of reference to the world and people. Introversion, to the Indian, is experiencing the world from the "looks within place," the power of intuition and introspection. Extroversion is the experience of illumination and enlightenment. The movement is from the outer world into the inner and back.

Some people's natural way of perceiving reality is through thinking, seeing things from the North, the place of wisdom and logic. Others see the world from a place of trust and innocence, the South, through their feeling function. Some are tuned into intuition, the power of the West. Others are more sensitive to fine details, to the illumination of the East.

Our most well-developed function can get us through life; but to individuate, to be a warrior, one must participate in the sacred marriage, the union of opposites. One must learn to dance with the powers of the four directions.

To move along the path toward wholeness, we must confront our projections, discover our shadow. The Indians say you must cast your shadow at your feet and learn to dance with your Shadow Chief.

Both Jung and the native way emphasize the existence and importance of the contra-sexual side of the psyche. Jung refers to the feminine energy as anima, the masculine as the animus. I am more comfortable with the images I get from using spirit and soul to describe these energies. Natives say there is a woman inside every man and a man inside every woman. Both stress the importance of knowing the inner man and woman and not passing that function onto an outer relationship.

The Indian's spiritual life was not separate from physical, social, and emotional development. Jung likewise connected the spiritual with the ordinary, science with magic, the night realm with the waking world. Both teach that individuation, the warrior's path, is a calling and a conscious commitment.

The dance between my Indian self and my Jungian self is complementary. When I get lost in the esoteric, intellectual aspect of Jung's work, the clear simplicity of the native way grounds me. I even find it easier to read and enjoy Jung's writings in the collected works when I'm grounded in my Indian self. Likewise, when a critical voice within begins to whisper how weird my Indian self is, the intellectual, conceptual, Swiss aspect of Jung and his writings ground me, and give me courage to continue my explorations.

I feel the interrelatedness of Jung, the Native American way, and my experience of life in my clinical practice. Recently a woman's emerging assertive spirit came to her as a pull to the mountains. As we followed the image over a period of time via dreams, daydreams, and discussions of what we know about mountains, she felt the spirit of the mountain. The mountain taught her of her firm, solid, essence. The mountain was grounded in the earth and reached to the sky. Then the woman felt free to explore the caverns of the mountain, the sharp rocky edges along with the brush and vegetation. Other women I work with use the image of being rooted in the earth to deal with the anxiety of moving their new growth into the outer world. The connections between personal experience, nature, and the archetypes arise in endless images which are teachers.

Another effect of my Jungian/Indian dance on my clinical practice and my personal life is a valuing of ritual. Now I find myself spontaneously imagining rites of passage as I listen to my patients or help my daughter Amy prepare for a piano recital or go away to camp for the first time. To illustrate: Yesterday Don, my husband/co-therapist, and I were working together with another husband and wife. Their family consists of a 13-year-old daughter whom the father sexually abused and a 9-year-old son who has only been told that Daddy is out of the home because of marital problems. The father legally can have no contact with the daughter. The husband and wife do not want to be separated. The mother was a victim of sexual abuse and has used denial to deal with the effects of incest on her. The daughter is rageful, terrified, and self-destructive. The brother is angry at the sister, intuiting that she is connected to father's absence and he is not being told the truth. The father is pressing us for a family session for which the daughter is not ready. We are getting ready to go on a 3-week vacation. What comes to me is a ritual that I describe. Within it is the prescription for change which must occur in each family member and within the system before the family can reunite as a new entity. When these goals are accomplished we will have a ritual acknowledging the old family with its shadow, recognizing the changes we have been effecting (the death and rebirth), and defining and celebrating the new individuals who make up the family. Individual and family therapy will continue to support the new life and confront the old when it starts to seep in.

The ritual I envision is as follows, I ask each family member to come up with two images. The first symbolizes the old self that is dying through the process of psychotherapy. The second is a symbol of the new self being birthed. The images are then given material form. Family members may draw their image, sculpt it with clay, or find a suitable representation in nature to house the spirit of the self. Each person speaks first to the dark spirit of the old self, banishes it, asserts his or her freedom from its control, and gives it up to either the earth or the fire for transformation. Then each person welcomes the spirit of their new self, again symbolized in material form. The symbols of the new selves which compose the new family system are placed in the center inner circle. We then bless these new beginnings and commit ourselves to their continual support and growth.

My Indian and Jungian dance is my experience of soul psychology. I live this dance in my daily life. Inherent in the word psychology is the task of the therapist—bringing into consciousness and manifestation the wisdom of the soul. Research into soul psychology follows the image of the Native American weaver. The Indian woman takes the wool from the animal, works it into thread, then weaves it into a pattern that includes symmetry and repetition. However, she always weaves in an irregular thread acknowledging the necessity of the soul's escape from the captivity of concept and form. The soul's dance is ever changing. To participate, we must learn to follow.

REFERENCES

Jung, C. G. (1960). The soul and death. In H. Read, M. Fordham, & G. Adler (Eds.) and R. Hull (Trans.), *The collected works of C. G. Jung* (Vol. 8, pp. 404-415). Princeton: Princeton University Press/Bollingen Series XX.

Storm, H. (1972). *Seven arrows.* New York: Ballentine Books.

von Franz, M. L. (1980). *Alchemy: An introduction to the symbolism and the psychology.* Toronto: Inner City Books.

Barbara Jo Brothers
Associate Editor of VOICES

But to the Vision Opposite in Space

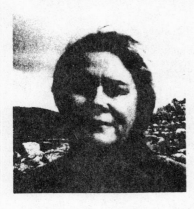

Barbara Jo Brothers is in private practice. She received her MSW from Tulane University in 1965. Since that time she has explored, and is still exploring, wide ranges and promising avenues toward the healing of the human psyche and soul, collectively and/or individually. Her interests flow toward the far horizons of who we are—and who we might become.

New Orleans, Louisiana 70115
3500 St. Charles Avenue

I debated with myself, I really wanted to not miss the solar eclipse. I have an intense fascination regarding astronomical matters. This was the first one of this nature to come my way.

And I was scheduled for Sally at 11. Cancel it and change the time? (Sally had very recently told me what she had not told the referring therapist . . . that she is subject to feeling suicidal when she gets depressed.) This was not a run-of-the-mill psychotherapy session. Sally, a very bright professional woman who had recently moved to my community to change careers, had confessed much deeper depression to me last week than she ever confided to her previous therapist. I had realized, to my growing dismay, that she was an ideal candidate, if one can use such terms in this sort of situation, for suicide. She was in a new city with no support system. I had not yet become aware that there was a *much* greater level of pathology afoot than first met the eye, but I already had an intuitive feeling that this woman required delicate handling.

So I sat through one of our initial sessions in the strange not quite so earthly light of the solar eclipse . . . and then the eerier midday darkening. Modern America was out observing a spectacular natural event. I was engaged already with the Force of Darkness that had eclipsed Sally a long time ago. In retrospect, it feels right to have been doing battle with such an element on such a day. Not that Sally herself paid any mind to this. Had I mentioned any of this to her, she would have replied with scorn, if she could have found words at all, for such flagrant disregard of modern science.

And that was part of the trouble for Sally as I saw it. It was both the trouble and her refuge. Her intelligence and ability to discipline her mind had saved her from the emotional wreckage of a desolate childhood where she was the least favored, born to a pair of old maids in spite of their having been physiologically and socially the correct juxtaposition of sexes.

At the point she was referred to me by a colleague from out of town, I was attending a series of weekend seminars, a part of Jean Houston's New York State based Mystery School, in which we were studying ancient mystery schools and ancient methods of healing. Sally came to me between two weeks in which the focus had been on the Jesus mystery, including Jesus' method of healing, integrated with the Eastern notions of energy and chakras. These two weekends dealt with the heart chakra. I have to confess I really didn't even know what a chakra was until that spring. In fact, I think I need to confess having had what I would have to call a Western prejudice about such notions. I missed the now old, "new" fad of Eastern religion/mysticism when it began to blossom.

Sally was well dressed and had a certain poise about her. She was obviously quite bright, having a Ph.D. in science. In fact, it came out that we shared the same alma mater for our undergraduate degrees and had been in the same graduating class years ago in another state. So I knew precisely *how* bright she had to be in order to obtain a degree in the sciences at that particular place and time. It took considerable left-brain organization as well as intelligence. As it turned out, I needed all this extra reason to feel connected to her. There was a terrible barrenness about Sally which fairly soon became much clearer. A terrible lonely barrenness which I saw stretching back through the '50s and back into the early '40s. I saw that loneliness that most of us don't know. The bone-deep loneliness, that crying from a cradle to an empty room loneliness, that loneliness born of being mechanically fed with abrupt hands and met by distracted eyes.

Sally, as she told her life story, told me soon about open heart surgery 2 years past and about the depression that went with it.

Of course, I thought. A broken, battered heart. All left brain, sustained by her intellect alone all these years . . . and the *heart* all wrong.

No heart beating right. That is what this woman needs, I have to reach that poor battered heart. (Virginia Satir on psychosomatic illness: The body says what the mouth won't.)

But *how?* She so distant, so rigid, so into reward only from her intellect.

Ironic, she had given up a university post to move to this city. "I got lonely," she said, "I was so isolated." She was looking for a new professional life. "I needed more," she said. I knew she did. I felt the aching loneliness, the isolation of a small town for a single woman getting older without the family structure in which that culture functions.

But all her self-esteem had always been based on work. There was nothing else in her life. No child, no lover, no friend. Only the work. Only the science. And she had at last become too emotionally drained to sustain her commitment to her own specific project. After the surgery, she had allowed it to be taken over by others.

So here she was, having hurled herself out of context; no job to tell her she had a place in the world. A new city, new faces, no support system. No habits or routines. Where had that kind of breaking-loose courage come from?

But she would give herself no credit, take no praise. No way to build her self-esteem that route, whether or not it spoke of courage to me. She could only tell me about her fear and anxiety of having no job now.

Sally had put all her eggs in the left-lobe basket and was a child of the puritan ethic. If she worked hard and produced something then she had a chance at justifying her existence. Hence her current abysmal depression: Her temporary job was ending and she had no permanent one beginning. So what was she alive for? What reason did she have to be on this earth?

Nor did Sally have any human beings in her life to balance that work-is-life idea in any way. She had no close friends either in the community to which she had moved or in the one she had left. She had thought once that she was in love, back when she was in graduate school, but she had chosen to focus on job opportunities after her graduation, leaving whatever was that possibility to remain "what might have been." So she had no lovers as well as no friends. Sally was 43, an age when empty dreams begin to come home to roost even for people with fuller lives. Nobody loved her; why was she alive?

That question was much harder for me to deal with. Sally was cold, judgmental, and rigid. Hardly the sort of person who draws warmth and concern. Her loneliness was of that ancient sort that had given up centuries ago so that she survived on her own desert island as if she were her own almost extinct tribe. Sally's heart had that sort of emptiness that has never known fullness. It did not surprise me when she told me that she had open heart surgery 2 years ago and had a weak heart. It was a metaphor as apt as our shared eclipse had been.

A session or two after the eclipse, Sally told me about cyanide tablets.

She had brought them home from the lab years ago in the event she ever felt the need to kill herself. I got colder chills than I have ever gotten while listening to any other body's suicidal ideation as I listened to her account.

I was beginning to have the uneasy feeling that a miracle was in order here, whether I liked it or not, and I had a pretty clear idea that I was all that stood between this woman and Death. I reflected back on the weekend seminar on healing. Having been reared in the Bible belt and within broadcast range of Oral Roberts, I grew up with a disdain that would match Sally's about this "non-scientific" stuff. Still, face-to-face with Sally, I was facing the conviction that she could well die within a few weeks if I didn't do something pretty convincing. This is the sort of person for whom a mental hospital can easily do nothing. She was not disorganized in her thinking. The weak heart would preclude electro-convulsive shock treatment (God forbid, but that is a course somebody might have considered taking); she was already taking an anti-depressant prescribed by some physician in New York whose name been given by a friend from 10 years back. There was no place to "send" her that was likely to be more effective than I would be.

I don't know whether the concept of synchronicity actually has validity or not, but I did have to consider the presence of a pattern here. If somebody had set out to design a living example of a "heart-chakra problem," Sally could not have been a more adequate embodiment. And I had so recently come from a weekend of learning about the healing nature of being in touch with the depth of one's own essence, about how to tap into one's own heart chakra for healing energy.

I got up from my chair, sat down beside Sally, put my arms around her and focused all my "energy"/concentration on my heart, her heart, my heart, her heart. I gathered in all the warmth I could find in my own, I beamed it as steadily and purely as I could into her. I did find that the effort itself seemed to energize me for more effort. I prayed. I *knew* I was standing between this woman and Death and I did *not* know whether the best I had to give her was going to be enough.

After that I did my standard suicide-prevention tact of getting an agreement from the patient to "call me first." Weeks went by and there was no change. In fact, there were days that seemed even worse. . . .

Then I got the call.

She was drunk although it was early afternoon, and she had the tablet in her hand, but she had promised me she would call. So she was calling.

What does a responsible therapist do at a time like that? If one does the legally correct thing, one could lose the patient. Even if I had been able to figure out a way to keep her on the phone and call the police at the same time, she would have been quite likely to swallow the tablet when she saw them at the door. I prayed some more and somehow talked her into coming in to see me the next morning instead. The next morning I had a psychiatrist friend poised in the next office with commitment papers. When Sally got there, she said she didn't feel so bad anymore. I began to breathe again. My friend put away all the papers.

More weeks went by and Sally continued to talk intermittently about the cyanide tablets. I continued to feel very uncomfortable and as if I was walking a tightwire with her in my arms. I had begun seeing her in late May. At that point, I had no idea that the fact that I planned to leave the country for several weeks in January would constitute a particular problem. As my trip grew closer, I began to be increasingly concerned about what I would do with Sally. I tried putting her in a group, which turned out to be a disaster. I had to admit to myself that I had underestimated her pathology and that she was considerably more than just "unsocialized." She wasn't somebody I could send to a colleague to "tide her over."

Then a very curious thing happened.

The effect on me was no less startling than if I had gone into a movie theater to see *Gone with the Wind* and suddenly found *Star Wars* immediately following the burning of Atlanta.

Sally had come in and begun her litany of I-can't-find-a-job (more than 2 months of unemployment had passed), why-am-I-alive, I-have-no-family-I've-done-nothing-with-my-life, looking as depressed as ever . . . and her appearance was even beginning to slip subtly. In the middle of the morass of depression, she said, "I met somebody this week. I think I like him," and almost immediately went back into the gloom. Next session she mentioned him again with the same back-to-the-bad immediately following. Within short weeks of my impending trip and only a few sessions later, she said, "Marvin asked me to marry him. I think I'm going to do it." Then went immediately back to why-am-I-alive, I-have-no-job, I have-done-nothing-with-my-life. In the ensuing session it was like a special-effects series of scenes in a visual-arts production. The Old Sally would be there, looking slightly disheveled in that disintegrating sort of way that goes with psychotic depression and presenting one reality so convincingly that part of me believed her. She was hopelessly "behind" in life; she'd made no success of her work; she'd created no family; she was hopeless. Then pieces of a completely different reality would start showing through, almost like a "whole" behind breaking-up pieces of a rigid image. "He wants to marry me. He wants a baby by me. He's the nicest man I ever knew."

I couldn't stand the incongruence. "Sally, both statements can't be true. You can't be hopelessly unlovable if there is somebody who is resolutely loving you." She had to agree to the logic of this. I was as reluctant as she was. In fact, it may have seemed even *less* believable to me than it did to her. But, sure enough, this person had showed up in what had been her empty life and was, *just by virtue of his presence,* turning her previous premises upside down. She could not say nobody had ever loved her, nobody had ever wanted her, it was hopeless to hope for anything different. He was right there, as close to the answer to a prayer as anything I've ever seen.

27

The week after I got back into the country after my trip, I attended her church wedding, white dress and all. The week before I left she'd decided maybe she shouldn't have those cyanide tablets lying around; her husband-to-be had a child by his previous marriage, there would be other people in the house.

I promise you all, I would not believe any of this if I had not been there, but it has been nearly a year now and I have not heard from her since. For want of anything better to call it, I have to call it therapeutic success. I make *no* pretense, however, that I can account for it.

> *Our moons may have a darker side than most,*
> *But to the Vision Opposite in space*
> *Be visible when light's reflected ghost*
> *Is in eclipse on earth's astonished face.*

(Brothers, 1963, p. 38)

REFERENCE

Brothers, R. L. (1963). Poem for Patricia. *Threescore and ten.* San Antonio: The Naylor Company.

James Hillman **Soul and Spirit**

James Hillman practices analysis, teaches, lectures, edits, and writes. He was Director of Studies at the C. G. Jung Institute in Zurich (1959-1969), Graduate Dean at the University of Dallas (1979-1980), Founding Fellow of the Dallas Institute of Humanities and Culture. He has given the Terry Lectures at Yale University; and held various visiting professorships at Syracuse, Yale, University of Chicago, etc. He is publisher and editor (since 1970) of SPRING Publications and its annual, *Spring*. His books include *The Myth of Analysis, The Dream and the Underworld, Inter Views, Freud's Own Cookbook* (with Charles Boer), as well as *Healing Fiction, Loose Ends, Emotion, Pan and the Nightmare,* and others. In 1981, Dr. Hillman was awarded the Medal of the Community of Florence, Italy, for his contribution to psychology deriving from the Italian Renaissance.

Box 412
Thompson, Connecticut 06277

In Suicide and the Soul *(1964) which is the first full-length modern psychology book to take up that nasty four letter word S O U L, there are some paragraphs (pp. 43-47) that tell what I mean by the word:*

Jung alone among the great psychologists refused to classify people into groups according to their sufferings. He has been charged with failing to provide a detailed and systematic theory of neurosis along with etiology and treatment. Is this really a failing? Perhaps it is his virtue to have alone recognized the gross inadequacy of only outside descriptions.

An analyst faces problems, and these problems are not merely classifiable behavioral acts, not medical categories of disease. They are above all experiences and sufferings, problems with an "inside." The first thing that the patient wants from an analyst is to make him aware of his suffering and to draw the analyst into his world of experience. Experience and suffering are terms long associated with soul. "Soul," however, is not a scientific term, and it appears very rarely in psychology today, and then usually with inverted commas as if to keep it from infecting its scientifically sterile surround. Soul cannot be accurately defined, nor is it respectable in scientific discussion as now understood. There are many words of this sort which carry meaning, yet which find no place in today's science. It does not mean that the references of these words are not real because scientific method fails or leaves them out. Nor does it mean that scientific method fails because it omits these words which lack operational definition. All methods have their limits; we need but keep clear what belongs where.

To understand soul we cannot turn to science for a description. Its meaning is best given by its context, and this context has already been partly stated. The root metaphor of the analyst's point of view is that human behavior is understandable because it has an inside meaning. The inside meaning is suffered and experienced. It is understood by the analyst through sympathy and insight. All these terms are the everyday empirical language of the analyst and provide the context for and are expressions of the analyst's root metaphor. Other words long associated with the word soul amplify it further: mind, spirit, heart, life, warmth, humanness, personality, individuality, intentionality, essence, innermost, purpose, emotion, quality, virtue, morality, sin, wisdom, death, God. A soul is said to be "troubled," "old," "disembodied," "immortal," "lost," "innocent," "inspired." Eyes are said to be soulful, for the eyes are "the mirror of the soul"; but one can be "soulless" by showing no mercy. Most "primitive" languages have elaborate concepts about animated principles which ethnologists have translated by "soul." For these peoples, from ancient Egyptian to modern Eskimo, soul is a highly differentiated idea referring to a reality of great impact. The soul has been imaged as the inner man, and as the inner sister or spouse, the place or voice of God within, as a cosmic force in which all humans, even all things living, participate, as having been given by God and thus divine, as conscience, as a multiplicity and as a unity in diversity, as a harmony, as a fluid, as fire, as dynamic energy, and so on. One can "search one's soul" and one's soul can be "on trial." There are parables describing possession of the soul by and sale of the soul to the Devil, of temptations of the soul, of the damnation and redemption of the soul, of development of the soul through spiritual disciplines, of journeys of the soul. Attempts have been made to localize the soul in specific body organs and regions, to trace its origin to sperm or egg, to divide it into animal, vegetable, and mineral components, while the search for the soul leads always into the "depths."

As well, arguments continue on the connection of the soul with the body: that they are parallel; that the soul is an epiphenomenon of the body, a sort of internal secretion; that the body is only the throbbing visibility of an immaterial form-giving soul; that their relation is irrational and synchronistic, coming and going, fading and waxing, in accordance with psychoid constellations; that there is no relation at all; that flesh is mortal and the soul eternal, reincarnating by karma through the aeons; that each soul is individual and perishable, while it is the body as matter which cannot be destroyed; that soul is only present in sentient bodies possible of consciousness; or, that souls, like monads, are present in all bodies as the psychic hierarchy of nature alive.

From the points of view of logic, theology, and science, these statements are to be proved and disputed. From the point of view of psychology, they are one and all true positions, in that they are statements about the soul made by the soul. They are the soul's description of itself in the language of thought (just as the soul images itself in contradictions and paradoxes in the language of poetry and painting). This implies that at different moments each of these statements reflects a phase of the body-soul relationship. At one time it is synchronistic where everything falls in place. At another time soul and body are so identified, as in toxic states or disease, that epiphenomenalism is the true position. Or at another time, the life-course of the body and soul are radically independent and parallel. We must then conclude that such statements about the soul reflect the state of soul of the one making the statement. They reveal the special bent of a person's own psyche-soma problem, a problem that seems unendingly bound up with psychology and the riddle of the soul, since it is this question—what have the body and soul to do with each other—that the soul is continually putting to us in philosophy, religion, art, and above all in the trials of daily life and death.

This exploration of the word shows that we are not dealing with something that can be defined; and therefore, "soul" is really not a concept, but a symbol. Symbols, as we know, are not completely within our control, so that we are not able to use the word in an unambiguous way, even though we take it to refer to that unknown factor which makes meaning possible, which turns events into experiences, and which is communicated in love. The soul is a deliberately ambiguous concept resisting all definition in the same manner as do all ultimate symbols which provide the root metaphors for the systems of human thought. "Matter" and "nature" and "energy" have ultimately the same ambiguity; so too have "life," "health," "justice," "society," and "God," which provide the symbolic sources for the points of view we have already seen. Soul is not more an obfuscation than other axiomatic first principles. Despite modern man's unease with the term, it continues to stand behind and influence the point of view of depth psychology in ways which many depth psychologists themselves might be surprised to discover.

What a person brings to the analytical hour are the sufferings of the soul; while the meanings discovered, the experiences shared, and the intentionality of the therapeutic process are all expressions of a living reality which cannot be better apprehended than by the root metaphor of psychology, psyche or soul.

The terms "psyche" and "soul" can be used interchangeably, although there is a tendency to escape the ambiguity of the word "soul" by recourse to the more biological, more modern "psyche." "Psyche" is used more as a natural concomitant to physical life, perhaps reducible to it. "Soul," on the other hand, has metaphysical and romantic overtones. It shares frontiers with religion.

*   *   *

This excursion on what I mean by soul was extended in Revisioning Psychology *(1975, pp. 67-70):*

By "soul" I mean, first of all, a perspective rather than a substance, a viewpoint toward things rather than a thing itself. This perspective is reflective; it mediates events and makes differences between ourselves and everything that happens. Between us and events, between the doer and the deed, there is a reflective moment—and soul-making means differentiating this middle ground.

It is as if consciousness rests upon a self-sustaining and imagining substrate—an inner place or deeper person or ongoing presence—that is simply there even when all our subjectivity, ego, and consciousness go into eclipse. Soul appears as a factor independent of the events in which we are immersed. Though I cannot identify soul with anything else, I also can never grasp it by itself apart from other things, perhaps because it is like a reflection in a flowing mirror, or like the moon which mediates only borrowed light. But just this peculiar and paradoxical intervening variable gives one the sense of having or being a soul. However intangible and indefinable it is, soul carries highest importance in hierarchies of human values, frequently being identified with the principle of life and even of divinity.

In another attempt upon the idea of soul I suggested that the word refers to that unknown component which makes meaning possible, turns events into experiences, is communicated in love, and has a religious concern. These four qualifications I had already put forth some years ago [see above]. I had begun to use the term freely, usually interchangeably with psyche (from Greek) and anima (from Latin). Now I am adding three necessary modifications. First, "soul" refers to the deepening of events into experiences; second, the significance soul makes possible, whether in love or in religious concern, derives from this special relation with death. And third, by "soul" I mean the imaginative possibility in our natures, the experiencing through reflective speculation, dream, image, and fantasy—that mode which recognizes all realities as primarily symbolic or metaphorical.

More on the excursion on the difference between psyche or soul on the one hand and spirit on the other:

Here we need to remember that the ways of the soul and those of the spirit only sometimes coincide and that they diverge most in regard to psychopathology. A main reason for my stress upon pathologizing is just to bring out the differences between soul and spirit, so that we end the widespread confusions between psychotherapy and spiritual disciplines. There is a difference between Yoga, transcendental meditation, religious contemplation and retreat, and even Zen, on the one hand, and the psychologizing of psychotherapy on the other. This difference is based upon a distinction between spirit and soul.

Today we have rather lost this difference that most cultures, even tribal ones, know and live in terms of. Our distinctions are Cartesian: between outer tangible reality and inner states of mind, or between body and a fuzzy conglomerate of mind, psyche, and spirit. We have lost the third, middle position which earlier in our tradition, and in others too, was the place of soul: a world of imagination, passion, fantasy, reflection, that is neither physical and material on the one hand, nor spiritual and abstract on the other, yet bound to them both. By having its own realm psyche has its own logic—psychology—which is neither a science of physical things nor a metaphysics of spiritual things. Psychological pathologies also belong to this realm. Approaching them from either side, in terms of medical sickness or religion's suffering, sin, and salvation, misses the target of soul.

But the threefold division has collapsed into two, because soul has become identified with spirit. This happens because we are materialists, so that everything that is not physical and bodily is one undifferentiated cloud; or it happens because we are Christians. Already in the early vocabulary used by Paul, pneuma or spirit had begun to replace psyche or soul. The New Testament scarcely mentions soul phenomena such as dreams, but stresses spirit phenomena such as miracles, speaking in tongues, prophecy, and visions.

Philosophers have tried to keep the line between spirit and soul by keeping soul altogether out of their works or assigning it a lower place. Descartes confined soul to the pineal gland, a little enclave between the opposing powers of internal mind and external space. More recently, Santayana has put soul down in the realm of matter and considered it an antimetaphysical principle. Collingwood equated soul with feeling and considered that psychology had no business invading the realm of thought and ideas. The spiritual point of view always posits itself as superior, and operates particularly well in a fantasy of transcendence among ultimates and absolutes.

Philosophy is therefore less helpful in showing the differences than is the language of the imagination. Images of the soul show first of all more feminine connotations. Psyche, in the Greek language, besides being soul, denoted a night-moth or butterfly and a particularly beautiful girl in the legend of Eros and Psyche. Our discussion in the previous chapter of the anima as a personified feminine idea continues this line of thinking. There we saw many of her attributes and effects, particularly the relationship of psyche with dream, fantasy, and image. This relationship has also been put mythologically as the soul's connection with the night world, the realm of the dead, and the moon. We still catch our soul's most essential nature in death experiences, in dreams of the night, and in the images of "lunacy."

The world of spirit is different indeed. Its images blaze with light, there is fire, wind, sperm. Spirit is fast, and it quickens what it touches. Its direction is vertical and ascending; it is arrow-straight, knife-sharp, powder-dry, and phallic. It is masculine, the active principle, making forms, order, and clear distinctions. Although there are many spirits, and many kinds of spirit, more and more the notion of "spirit" has come to be carried by the Apollonic archetype, the sublimations of higher and abstract disciplines, the intellectual mind, refinements, and purifications.

We can experience soul and spirit interacting. At moments of intellectual concentration or transcendental meditation, soul invades with natural urges, memories, fantasies, and fears. At times of new psychological insights or experiences, spirit would quickly extract a meaning, put them into action, conceptualize them into rules. Soul sticks to the realm of experience and to reflections within experience. It moves indirectly in circular reasonings, where retreats are as important as advances, preferring labyrinths and corners, giving a metaphorical sense to life through such words as close, near, slow, and deep. Soul involves us in the pack and welter of phenomena and the flow of impressions. It is the "patient" part of us. Soul is vulnerable and suffers; it is passive and remembers. It is water to the spirit's fire, like a mermaid who beckons the heroic spirit into the depths of passions to extinguish its certainty. Soul is imagination, a cavernous treasury—to use an image from St. Augustine—a confusion and rightness, both. Whereas spirit chooses the better part and seeks to make all One. Look up, says spirit, gain distance; there is something beyond and above, and what is above is always superior.

They differ in another way: spirit is after ultimates and it travels by means of a *via negativa*. "Neti, neti," it says, "not this, not that." Strait is the gate, and only first or last things will do. Soul replies by saying, "Yes, this too has a place, may find its archetypal significance, belongs in a myth." The cooking vessel of the soul takes in everything, everything can become soul; and by taking into its imagination any and all events, psychic space grows.

I have drawn apart soul and spirit in order to make us feel the differences, and especially to feel what happens to soul when its phenomena are viewed from the perspective of spirit. Then it seems, the soul must be disciplined, its desires harnessed, imagination emptied, dreams forgotten, involvements dried. For soul, says spirit, cannot know, neither truth, nor law, nor cause. The soul is fantasy. The thousand pathologizings that soul is heir to by its natural attachments to the ten thousand things of life in the world shall be cured by making soul into an imitation of spirit. The "imitatio Christi" was the classical way; now there are other models, gurus from the Far East or Far West, who if followed to the letter, put one's soul on a spiritual path which supposedly leads to freedom from pathologies. Pathologizing, so says spirit, is by its very nature confined only to soul; only the psyche can be pathological, as the word psychopathology attests. There is no "pneumopathology," and as one German tradition has insisted, there can be no such thing as mental illness ("Geisteskrankheit"), for the spirit cannot pathologize. So there must be spiritual disciplines for the soul, ways in which soul shall conform with models enunciated for it by spirit.

But from the viewpoint of the psyche the humanistic and Oriental movement upward looks like repression. There may well be more psychopathology actually going on while transcending than while being immersed in pathologizing. For any attempt at self-realization without full recognition of the psychopathology that resides, as Hegel said, inherently in the soul is in itself pathological, an exercise in self-deception. Such self-realization turns out to be a paranoid delusional system, or even a kind of charlatanism, the psychopathic behavior of an emptied soul.

REFERENCES

Hillman, J. (1964). *Suicide and the soul*. New York: Harper & Row.
Hillman, J. (1975). *Re-visioning psychology*. New York: Harper & Row.

COMMENT

Hillman has shined the dark light of his vision on soul for two decades and then some. As Jung was not a Jungian, Hillman is neither Jungian or Hillmanian. Ego is not an important part of his message.

I recently had the experience of a seminar with James Hillman and Patricia Berry, husband and wife, teachers and soul-mates. The subject was Images and Symbols in Dreams and Fairy tales. The setting was Casa Maria, a convent turned residential seminar center, in Santa Barbara. For 5 days, 75 of us immersed ourselves in the images of the dreams and fairy tales selected by James and Pat, or volunteered by the participants. Imagine that luxury! I felt like one of the wealthiest men in the world.

Hillman and Berry teach, as Jung did, that soul communicates through images and that images stand for what they are. The fox in the dream or fairy tale stands for a fox. We are to learn from the fox the ways of the fox. We are not to fall victim to the ego's attempts to redefine the fox in our own image and likeness.

Reading Hillman has always turned me inside out and upside down. I have spent a great deal of my life in the underworld, but was always trying to take the light of the upperworld, the sun, ego consciousness, with me to ease my terror. Watching and listening to Hillman, I was able to let go and enter the shadowy realm illumined by lunar light, by reflected light, with soul consciousness.

What a relief. Everything is as it is. I cannot possibly understand anything. I (ego) can only experience and learn.

Take Hillman for a guide. It's a trip you'll never forget.

DONALD LATHROP, M.D.

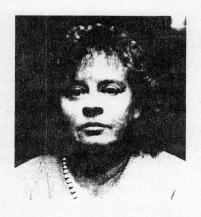

Janet Dallett

When the Spirits Come Back*

I was punished for being a Kindergarten tattletale, which effectively silenced me for almost half a century. When I became an analyst, professional sanctions and esoterica surrounding the notion of secrecy conveniently supported my childhood neurosis. At 52, I feel entitled to begin to be who I am, a born tattletale, just like the teacher said. This paper is the beginning. Some facts, including my home town, have been altered to protect Sarah.

c/o Karen Gibson
111 West Curling Drive
Boise, Idaho 83702

The American presents a strange picture: a European with Negro behavior and an Indian soul. He shares the fate of all usurpers of foreign soil. Certain Australian primitives assert that one cannot conquer foreign soil, because in it there dwell strange ancestor-spirits who reincarnate themselves in the newborn. There is a great psychological truth in this. The foreign land assimilates its conqueror. . . . Thus, in the American, there is a discrepancy between conscious and unconscious that is not found in the European, a tension between an extremely high conscious level of culture and an unconscious primitivity. . . . Alienation from the unconscious and from its historical conditions spells rootlessness. That is the danger that lies in wait for the conqueror of foreign lands, and for every individual who . . . loses touch with the dark, maternal, earthy ground of his being.

C. G. JUNG (1961, p. 248)

This is Sarah's story but it is also mine. I met Sarah late in 1984. A year and a half earlier I left behind a busy analytical psychology practice in Los Angeles, along with teaching and other professional responsibilities at the C. G. Jung Institute there, and moved to Seal Harbor, a small town in the Pacific Northwest. I had no plans. I put aside preconceptions about what my life would be and waited, listening for the inner and outer voices that would tell me what might be required of me here. I walked a lot; watched my dreams; noticed my thoughts and fantasies; and talked with many people, paying attention to whose paths crossed mine, who attracted me, how I was moved to spend my time when I could do anything I chose.

My last year in Los Angeles had been a nightmare of growing disillusion with professional life. I cared about the psyche, about dreams, about people, but found myself increasingly enmeshed in considerations

---

* Published with the permission of Sarah Petrovici, a pseudonym.

of status and power that had nothing to do with my deeper concerns. In fact, the more "successful" I became, the less able I felt to serve life or soul. More than once I dreamed that my environment was filled with poison. Soon after dreaming of a funeral at the Jung Institute, I decided to leave.

Now, with unlimited time and space for the first time in many years, it was not long before I began to experience the impact of what is buried in the earth of this country. Without knowing at first what affected me so deeply, I was touched by aspects of Native American tribal consciousness that appeared to seep through the soles of my feet. While talking with a psychologist friend one day, I "saw" behind his eyes an immense Indian chief, gazing at me with longing, yearning to be set free from imprisonment in an alien white body. The same week I noticed the designation "Redman's Cemetery" on a local map and spent several days searching for it, convinced that I would find something of great importance, but at that location were only traditional, marble headstones with names like McGuire, O'Meara, Larson, and Scott. Confused, I looked at a different map and found this same spot labeled "Rectman's Cemetery."

A month later a visiting psychic told me she saw Indians in my house and in the surrounding forest. Still later, a mediumistic friend dreamed that she met me on the street and saw earth on my face. I looked, she said, like an old Indian woman.

I remembered the dream that my student Joseph had told me soon after he dropped out of the analyst training program. He was working on an archeological dig in his dream, apparently alone, not seeing much of what was going on at first, only a piece of bone here, a shard there. As the dream went on, however, he became aware that others were digging too, in many different places not necessarily visible from where he stood. By the end of the dream he had been given the perspective to see the scope of the project in which he was involved, the excavation of the skeleton of an enormous animal that extended from one coast to the other. Even at that time I wondered if the animal buried between the coasts of this continent might be connected to Native American consciousness.

Responding to the hints I was given, I began to learn what I could about the people who first occupied this land, a subject of previous indifference. I spent hours in anthropological museums and hiked for many miles to experience the power spots people told me about when they learned of my interest. Meanwhile I read, finding out what I could about native ways of life, legends, art, and healing practices. I was struck by the respect for truth, for nature, and for the heart in what I learned of the tribal consciousness that was here before it collided with European values. I discovered in it a humility and capacity to live with other human beings that is profoundly lacking in the superimposed culture. I saw in native ways an integration of both healing and art into life, a refusal to cut apart threads that are woven together simply and naturally into unified patterns of living.

Immersion in this land and in the material it opened me to took me inexorably deeper into mistrust of the profession that had previously contained me. Although my consciousness was too developed just to imitate Native American practices, neither could I continue naively to emulate the professional forms I had been taught. Six weeks after moving I resigned from the professional organization to which I belonged. Two months later I had a terrifying dream:

"I awake knowing that sometime in the night, somewhere the Bomb has dropped. I have been near the epicenter and am contaminated with radiation. A few people are reaching toward me, wanting to touch me. Most avoid me, knowing that if they touch me they will be irreversibly contaminated."

Following this dream I found myself unexpectedly and precipitously terminating the analytical relationship I had maintained for several years with a good friend and colleague. What erupted between us then also virtually severed our personal and collegial connections.

Suddenly I was without strong professional connections, more or less alone with a terrible need to break old molds, along with the terrible guilt entailed. Seeking friends with whom I could talk about the psyche, I found more psychological depth, good instincts, and emotional support among "ordinary people," particularly artists of various persuasions, than among members of my own profession. I began to value the human condition in a new way and to deplore the exaggerated sense of specialness that adheres to the professional practitioner. Slowly absorbing my radioactivity, I reflected about the separation that exists between life and the practice of analysis.

Professional analysis carries the bias of the Judeo-Christian era, wherein a great deal of attention has been paid to the tree of knowledge but the tree of life has fallen into the unconscious. That is to say, the profession values understanding but may not necessarily promote the process of living. All too often analysis "understands" life out of existence before it has a chance to happen. Many of the forms of analysis protect the analyst from certain hard things, but do not necessarily serve either the patient or the psyche. Instead, they foster an arrogance of professionalism that must be left behind if we are to grow beyond the isolation of power and the power of isolation into the eros hidden in the human condition.

For example, professional sanctions against maligning our colleagues serve an important function up to a point, but are too often carried far beyond that point and used to protect analyst prestige inappropriately. In the process, an enormous split is created in the collective psyche of the profession. On the one hand, being human we *do* gossip, but when we gather together in professional groups we pretend we have not said or heard the things we have. Therefore, many matters of importance are discussed behind backs but are never confronted openly. In addition to creating whited sepulchres, this strange pretense deprives us of healthy ways to defuse and to integrate the things we dislike about each other, and of a social function that would otherwise help to control conditions like psychopathy and psychological inflation that are undesirable for both the individual and the group.

The Kwakiutl Indians brought the human need to gossip into the realm of the sacred, providing ceremonially for its vital psychological and social functions. My patient Colette connected me to this information through a dream in which she was given a small box containing, of all things, a mouth! The image quite mystified me until I saw an exhibit of Kwakiutl masks in Seattle. There in a glass case was Colette's dream mouth, a carved wooden object called Talking Mouth. In Kwakiutl custom only certain people have the privilege of the mouth which, held between the owner's teeth, represents the right to speak about, "call down," or criticize other people publicly. The remarks themselves are made by a speaker standing beside the wearer of the mouth. Offense may not be taken at the comments of anyone who wears Talking Mouth (Molm, 1972, p. 52). The custom would serve professional psychology well!

Some version of the Nootka Indian practice of clowning would also add immensely to professional life. In a short story, Anne Cameron (1981) describes the clown through the eyes of Granny, an old Nootka woman:

> A clown was like a newspaper, or a magazine, or one of those people who write an article to tell you if a book or a movie is worth botherin' with. They made comment on everythin', every day. all the time. If a clown thought that what the tribal council was gettin' ready to do was foolish, why the clown would just show up at the council and imitate every move every one of the leaders made. Only the clown would imitate it in such a way every little wart on that person would show, every hole in their idea would suddenly look real big. . . . Everythin' you did, the clown did. And nobody would ever dare blow up at the clown! If you did that, well, you were just totally shamed. A clown didn't do what a clown did to hurt you or make fun of you or be mean, it was to show you what you looked like to other people. . . .
>
> If you thought every word you spoke was gospel, the clown would just stroll along behind you babblin' away like a simple-mind or a baby. Every up and down of your voice, the clown's voice

would go up and down until you finally heard what an ass you were bein'. Or maybe you had a bad temper and yelled a lot when you got mad, or hadn't learned any self control or somethin' like that. Well, the clown would just have fits. Every time you turned around there'd be the clown bashin' away with a stick on the sand or kickin' like a fool at a big rock, or yellin' insults back at the gulls, and just generally lookin' real stupid.

We need our clowns, and we used 'em to help us all learn the best ways to get along with each other. Bein' an individual is real good, but sometimes we're so busy bein' individuals we forget we gotta live with a lot of other people who all got the right to be individuals too, and the clowns could show us if we were gettin' a bit pushy, or startin' to take ourselves too serious. Wasn't nothin' sacred to a clown. Sometimes a clown would find another clown taggin' along behind, imitatin', and then the first one knew that maybe somethin' was gettin' out of hand, and maybe the clown was bein' mean or usin' her position as a clown to push people around and sharpen her own axe for her own reasons. But mostly the clowns were very serious about what they did. (pp. 109-110)

I look forward, probably with more optimism than is warranted, to a time when we may all be freer to speak openly about one another and even to mock each other a little, clown style. What we see in others may hurt, but if spoken and received openly it need not injure. There is no point in thinking we are too important to let our shortcomings be seen. They are quite visible anyway, often to everyone but ourselves. We who most need the humanizing effects of what others see, because professional status gives us so much power, are just the ones whom professionalism unfortunately protects. The doctor-patient archetype does, after all, have two poles that are bound together within the healthy person. The analyst who identifies too much with "doctor," forgetting that he or she is also "patient," all too often fails to constellate the psyche's healing power in outer-world patients because of an unconscious need to have them remain sick.

Rooted in European tradition, psychoanalytic forms, including the Jungian, have a precarious existence on this soil, unconnected as they are to the native psyche. The psyche behaves as if it wants to bridge the gap, not to regress to so-called primitive forms but to decrease the disparity between analysis as it is practiced and life as it is here. Seeking to serve that impulse, 6 months after moving to the Pacific Northwest I began to work with five carefully selected patients under conditions designed to push the limits of traditional models, and specifically to experiment with integrating the work more deeply with everyday life.

For each of these five people I set aside a full afternoon or evening rather than a 50-minute hour, working until we agree that we have gone as far as we can with the material at hand. Sessions run from one to four or more hours, depending on the person, the material, and how each of us feels on a particular day. The people I picked to work with in this way all know each other and are also either my friends or people whose friendship I would not hesitate to seek. Except when there has been a special reason to do so, I have not promised these people a totally confidential analytic relationship. As in any human connection, more harm is sometimes done by keeping silent than by telling the right person the right thing at the right time, and I have found it important to explore the parameters of this dimension of psychological work. I have charged some of these people no money at all, but arranged for barter on a straight hour-for-hour basis, whether the trade be housecleaning, art, or medical help. When it has been important to charge some money for psychological reasons, I have kept the amounts small.

More than the usual amount of care, ethical sensitivity, psychological honesty, and inner strength is called upon to deal with the human problems that arise from such work. Neither participant has much room to hide, and many matters are brought to light that would never be touched under a stricter doctor-patient procedure. I have more than once longed for the relative personal safety of the old forms.

As I have grown more comfortable with the guilt of breaking professional rules, and have deepened into what is demanded of work that is more in tune with native aspects of the psyche, I have simultaneously been woven into the fabric of this community. In the weaving, I have begun to be conscious of the complexity of community in the depths of the psyche, wherein old patterns are brought into relation with the new in an amazing intertwining of synchronicities and connections. Threads were severed and the pattern badly obscured so long as I sat with patients only in my office, speaking to no one of what I saw there, cutting and labeling and handing down *ex cathedra* pronouncements about shadow, animus and anima projection, transference and countertransference, taking everything back to the ego as if there were no world out there, tearing the fabric so badly I often missed it completely, missed my patients' lives and my own, didn't get the picture at all, missed the whole show!

Some of the things that happened as I began to be part of this community are at least another story, maybe several. But this is Sarah's story and I want to introduce her to you. I met Sarah my second September in Seal Harbor, just before the spirits came back.

The Indians say that in spring and summer the Redman is involved in practical aspects of life. That is when he fishes, gathers berries, and makes whatever preparations he must to sustain himself in this climate. The spirits are away then, in the underworld, doing whatever they do there. In autumn, around the time of the equinox but not precisely then, they come back into this world. Then the Redman goes into his long-house and tells stories, dances spirit dances, gathers songs and poems, lives with the spirits all winter long while the bears hibernate.

When the spirits arrive you know it. The winds come and the tourists go home and the air is alive with *something*. The first time it happened I began the work I have just told you about. This time, my second autumn, I wanted to paint again. All the artists I knew said, "Don't take lessons, just paint," but I felt insecure. My painting is not professional, not "painterly," so I looked for a teacher. Someone told me that Sarah gives a good class. I like her work, and one day in September I telephoned her.

Something peculiar happened. After I identified myself and made my request, there was a long silence. Then Sarah began to talk. She must have talked for 20 minutes without a pause. On the face of it she was telling me why she wasn't going to give another class, but I had the eerie feeling that she had found her way into my head. She spoke of matters that were on my mind, about the problems inherent in living in a small community and being a professional person at the same time.

As abruptly as she had begun talking she stopped. There was another silence while I tried to think what to say. Then she asked, "Are you a *trained* Jungian analyst?" I assured her that I am.

"In that case," she said, "I might like to arrange a trade with you."

I said, "Oh. Then let's meet and talk about it."

We did not talk about it. We made no formal arrangement. For almost 4 months we met at roughly 2-week intervals, as the spirit moved, and talked about whatever came up. Sometimes we met at my house, sometimes hers, sometimes at a restaurant. Occasionally Katy, her infant daughter, was with her and sometimes her husband, Sam.

Sarah showed me slides of her work, critiqued mine, talked with me about the psychological significance of color. She suggested books for me to read and I offered some to her. Gradually she told me about herself. As her story unfolded I became aware of what had drawn her to me.

Before her move to Seal Harbor in 1981, Sarah lived near Mount St. Helens. One day she began to feel her inner world falling apart. Growing more and more disturbed as the days passed, she and the mountain erupted almost simultaneously. It was Helen's first eruption, Sarah's fourth. Against a backdrop of falling ash, gas-masked people, and impassable roads, her friends tried to find help for Sarah while she experienced herself almost splitting apart as she stood on the earth and tried to hold the moon in its orbit.

The discrepancy between the archetypal feminine spirit (moon) and the reality of Sarah's life as a woman (earth) was too great for her psyche to bear. Like so many women in our time, she became a piece of the ground on which this split tried to heal, forming a bridge between the earth and the great goddess of the moon who now, becoming autonomous, refuses to stay any longer in her ancient orbit.

Eventually Sarah was hospitalized for the fourth time since the age of 19. In the hospital she felt invaded, depersonalized, denied permission to do the work she felt she must do: preventing the earth and the moon from flying totally apart, holding the feminine archetype in some semblance of connection to life. "If only," she mused, "my friends hadn't been so frightened. I was all right. I had to do what I was doing. I wish they could have just understood and supported me in it. Instead they distanced themselves and assumed my language was of no significance to them."

She remembered one doctor who was kind to her and seemed to understand what was happening. Only one. When she saw a terrifying presence and asked him to do something about it, he knew enough to stand between her and it. She was grateful for the simple gesture that took her reality seriously.

"It happens about every 5 years," she told me.

"When did you say was the last time?"

"1980."

It was not hard for me to figure out. Now almost 39, Sarah was approaching another break. When I asked if she thought that was so, she changed the subject.

Our next few meetings were punctuated by Sarah's more or less indirect questions, designed to discover my attitudes about psychosis and particularly about hospitalization. I told her that I had, on occasion, worked with psychotic episodes outside the hospital, when light medication could be arranged and a family member was willing to carry 24-hour responsibility. In the past I had insisted on hospitalization only twice. In both cases the men had guns and threatened to use them, one on himself, one on someone else.

Later she asked directly, "What would you do if I called on you the next time it happens to me?" I laughed. I didn't really know in advance. "I suppose," I said, "I would ask you what you were experiencing and take it from there." I showed her John Perry's (1974) book, *The Far Side of Madness,* and told her of attitudes I share with him, that some psychoses constitute the psyche's attempt to heal itself, that hallucinations, delusions, and so-called bizarre ideation are like dreams which, if properly understood and integrated, carry a process of development rather than ultimate disintegration. I expressed the hope that if such process could happen in the right way, it might not have to repeat

The dynamic of psychosis manifests primitive levels of the psyche that polite contemporary society has all but buried. Specific content may be very modern, including images of interplanetary war and nuclear holocaust. But the process, the pull to madness itself, is very old. It is the pull to the spirit world that finds so little legitimate space in our materialistic culture. The psychotic's task is exactly the same as that of the analyst, to connect this world with the other. The Native American mind knows enough to give special status to what ours labels psychosis. In it may lie the call and initiation of shaman and healer.

Sarah and I had no contract, not even a verbal agreement, but I felt bound by my implicit promise to her. The evening of December 30, 1984, she paid me a visit. With her she brought a large brown paper bag filled with books, and an uncharacteristically decisive manner. She emptied the books on the floor, 16 novels by the same author. This man, she explained, had raped her when she was 19 years old, and now she was going to turn him in. She had compiled a dossier on him from his writings. Something about the way she spoke of it puzzled me. I remembered that she was first hospitalized at the age of 19. Clearly she *had* been raped at that time, but was it a literal, outer-world rape or had something else happened to her that she could only describe adequately as rape? I felt uncertain.

Suddenly, in mid-sentence, she put the books back into their bag, took a deep breath, leaned back and began to talk in a different way. Clearly and without pausing she told me first about her mother's murder, when Sarah was six, shot by a lover who then committed suicide. Next she described a series of difficult relationships with men, culminating in her first marriage. She had felt misunderstood, betrayed, and abandoned in each situation, her inner experience and feelings rejected or ignored. Finally she told, in detail, about each of her four hospital experiences. Having finished her recital she stood up to leave. I observed that the rapist had taken many forms in her life. She nodded and left with her bag of books.

I remembered Jung's (1961) description of his meeting with Ochwiay Biano, chief of the Taos Pueblo, wherein are etched many images of civilization's rapists:

> "See," Ochwiay Biano said, "how cruel the whites look. Their lips are thin, their noses sharp, their faces furrowed and distorted by folds. Their eyes have a staring expression, they are always seeking something. What are they seeking? The whites always want something; they are always uneasy and restless. We do not know what they want. We do not understand them. We think that they are mad."

I asked him why he thought the whites were all mad. "They say that they think with their heads," he replied. "Why of course. What do you think with?" I asked him in surprise.

"We think here," he said, indicating his heart.

I fell into a long meditation. For the first time in my life, so it seemed to me, someone had drawn for me a picture of the real white man. It was as though until now I had seen nothing but sentimental, prettified color prints. This Indian had struck our vulnerable spot, unveiled a truth to which we are blind. I felt rising within me like a shapeless mist something unknown and yet deeply familiar. And out of this mist, image upon image detached itself; first Roman legions smashing into the cities of Gaul, and the keenly incised features of Julius Caesar, Scipio Africanus, and Pompey. I saw the Roman eagle on the North Sea and on the banks of the White Nile. Then I saw St. Augustine transmitting the Christian creed to the Britons on the tips of Roman lances, and Charlemagne's most glorious forced conversions of the heathen; then the pillaging and murdering bands of the Crusading armies. With a secret stab I realized the hollowness of that old romanticism about the Crusades. Then followed Columbus, Cortes, and the other conquistadors who with fire, sword, torture, and Christianity came down upon even these remote pueblos dreaming peacefully in the Sun, their Father. I saw, too, the people of the Pacific islands decimated by firewater, syphilis, and scarlet fever carried in the clothes the missionaries forced on them.

It was enough. What we from our point of view call colonization, missions to the heathen, spread of civilization, etc., has another face—the face of a bird of prey seeking with cruel intentness for distant quarry—a face worthy of a race of pirates and highwaymen. All the eagles and other predatory creatures that adorn our coats of arms seem to me apt psychological representatives of our true nature. (pp. 247-249)

Yes, I thought, that is the rapist. That is what Whiteman consciousness does to the primitive psyche.

The following Saturday, January 5, Sarah's husband, Sam, Katy in his arms, knocked on my door and asked if we could talk. He was disturbed by the way Sarah was acting and wanted me to help him relate to it. He knew she had had some psychotic episodes, but he had been married to her less than 5 years and had no idea what to expect. They were leaving that night for a ski trip at Mount Rainier, and Sam hoped the wildness of the mountain would calm Sarah. I agreed that it might, but felt uneasy and urged him to call me if he needed to.

The next night the telephone rang. I talked with Sam, with Sarah, with Sam again. Then I wrote in my journal:

"Sarah Petrovici has crossed over. Sam stopped here Saturday to indicate his concern that this might be happening. They have been on a ski trip since. Tonight about 10:15 Sam called from a phone booth in the ski area and told me Sarah was having a hard time. When I talked with her she said Sam's father was standing in the middle of the road with cars whizzing past, in terrible danger (a hallucination). I asked her what kind of man he is, and she described *the most* wonderful, stable human being. I said, 'So it's terribly scary to have him in such danger.' She said yes. I asked if she wanted to come home, She said, 'definitely!' Sam asked if it could wait until morning and she said ok. When I asked if I could do anything more for her tonight she said, 'Can you assure me safe passage? There have been a few problems. . . .' I hesitated. How could I be sure? Then I said I thought I could assure her that. She sounded relieved. I will see her at 10:30 tomorrow morning."

I deluded myself that I would write in my journal every day throughout the process, keeping a record of the most important psychological material. In fact, this was the last entry in my journal for several weeks. It took all my energy simply to stay afloat.

That night I dreamed:

> I pass by David's office and stop in. There is a packed suitcase in the middle of the floor and the place is a mess. I realize that Sarah Petrovici went to see him professionally once or twice long ago, before I knew her, but she was dissatisfied and doesn't trust him. I leave David's office and go to see Sarah. She is doing very well, almost fully recovered from her psychotic episode, in much better shape than I had imagined.

Sarah's appearance in my dream revealed and clarified my inner connection with her. David is an outstanding analyst who works in a traditional manner, but not too rigidly so. He is bright, creative, competent, and kind, a living image of the ideal psychotherapist. In the outer world Sarah had never seen him, but *I* had been his patient for a time and the Sarah within me had not been satisfied. Unrelieved light, beauty, order, truth, goodness, reason, and moderation were inadequate to heal the primitive, creative woman.

In case I should forget, the dream reminded me that in my psyche the healing archetype can no longer be carried by the traditional white, masculine analytical model, no matter how perfectly the work may be done, because it is too separated from the wounded one, too disidentified from the wildly irrational, creative, primitive psyche. A mess, the office of the traditional analyst is ready to be left.

Coming as it did at this moment, on the brink of Sarah's break, the dream gave me clear and welcome warning not to fall back into old professional ways. She would not find her sanity in "David's office." That the dream Sarah was doing very well encouraged me also to trust her outer-world counterpart's strength to achieve safe passage.

46

Sam and Sarah did not reach home on schedule the next morning. Scenery whizzing past the moving car was more than Sarah could bear, and they spent most of the day stopped at a friend's house in the woods some distance from Seal Harbor. Responding to Sam's call, I found my way there, knocked on the door and walked in, feeling a little like Goldilocks. Sarah lay on a couch with her eyes closed. I said, "Hi, Sarah." Without opening her eyes she said firmly, "I will speak with no one but the Pope." And so it began.

Later that day Sarah pushed me away and ran about the room screaming, "Tabu, tabu, tabu! I am tabu! Don't touch me. I am contaminated." My dream of the Bomb came back to me. I said, "No. You are not tabu. I want to touch you. You don't have to carry it all by yourself." We worked on decontamination rituals repeatedly during the days that followed.

I did little to intervene in the process in Sarah's psyche, beyond offering to help carry her contamination and using very small doses of antipsychotic medication. That afternoon she was able to go on to her own house. I telephoned some friends and asked if they would help by being with Sarah a few hours each day. They, in turn, called people they knew. Before it was over, 25 community members in addition to her family had become involved. As long as it was necessary, Sarah had at least two people with her 24 hours a day. After 5 days she announced, "There is too much energy in this room. Some of you will have to leave." The "staff" was reduced accordingly. In a few more days she was able to manage her life again without a lot of extra help.

At the beginning, things happened too fast for me to give even brief instructions to most of the people who appeared at the door to be with Sarah. When there was opportunity to communicate I said only a little: 1) Sarah is in an all-right space. Try not to be afraid of it. Fear is not good for her. 2) Be yourself as fully as you can. If you need to protect yourself, either physically or emotionally, do it. 3) Do whatever you can to understand what Sarah is trying to say and where she is at any given moment, without trying to change it. 4) Sarah's task is to build a bridge between this world and the world where she is. If you see any way to help her with that, do it.

Sarah's approval was required before anyone who volunteered or was asked to help was permitted to spend time with her. She knew immediately who would be good for her, and most were a particular breed of cat. For the first time I became aware of specific qualities of the counterculture that came of age during the sixties. The Vietnam war, direct and indirect experiences of psychedelic drugs, and the overriding chaos of that time left many human beings now in their 30s and 40s deeply wounded. Some, of course, have covered up the damage and successfully identified with the cultural norms of their parents. Others are hopelessly lost. It is a third group of whom I speak. They have remained close to their wounds without making woundedness a virtue, and are thereby blessed with singular compassion and a fundamental knowledge and trust of the primitive psyche lacking to most of us who are older. These were Sarah's companions through her most vulnerable time. Insofar as possible we protected her from the impact of people too unconscious of their own wounds, too identified with "health."

For my part, I struggled daily with the "David" in me, who dared not trust Sarah's process and wanted to yield to inner and outer pressures to hospitalize her, to administer heavier doses of drugs, or to try in other ways to save her from her experience. I was at moments shocked and frightened by the extremes to which her psychosis took her, how far away she went from this world. What if "something happened"? What if she hurt herself, or committed suicide, or had an accident, or never came out of it at all? In this small community, where everyone sees everything, I would surely be burned as a witch!

This is the crux. There was never serious doubt in my mind about the best treatment for Sarah, but in choosing the best for her I put myself at risk. Those who know and can activate the healing power of nature draw ancient archetypes to themselves. Whiteman civilization and healing have for centuries flexed muscles of ego control, trying to gain power over nature. Anyone who learns to cooperate with nature in the Redman way stirs old hatreds, arousing the inadequately buried fear that nature remains bigger than we are and will ultimately get us all, despite our attempts to subdue her.

This is why Wolfe, one of Sarah's companions, stopped her work as a midwife several years ago. Unable to gain the cooperation of the medical establishment, she was threatened with jail if she continued midwifery. The same instincts and knowledge that had served her well as midwife made Wolfe the ideal facilitator of Sarah's process. She immediately identified it as labor, fraught with pain and possibly danger, but seeking its own natural goal. Bringing to psychological birth the same attitudes she had in the past brought to physical birth, she quietly took charge of replacing burned-out volunteers while constantly supporting Sarah in whatever she needed to do.

Images of giving birth and of being born were daily occurrences for Sarah. Many other themes recurred, including the search for her mother, interplanetary war, nuclear contamination, prayers and rituals to Odin and later to Ra, a probe of her cells to discover the genetic secret that would save mankind, a research project the Indians were going to do on the Whiteman.

One day she asked me, "Did you know there are all these little fishes in the underworld?"

In touching Sarah we were all drawn into her inner space and were in turn touched and connected to the deepest parts of ourselves, the stuff of mysticism, creativity, and madness, all three. Much of my time was best spent talking with the volunteers, trying to help them, and me, understand and integrate what we were experiencing. Until the intensity of her process slowed, the only thing I could do for Sarah directly was to avoid blocking her way. I visited her several times a day in order to keep myself informed. Otherwise I simply tried to keep one foot in this world and to help her helpers do the same.

As the days passed I became aware that contamination by Sarah's process carried healing for everyone who participated in it, each person in a slightly different way. In addition, it contained the possibility for healing something larger than the sum of individuals, a malaise in the community among us. In *The Four-Gated City* Doris Lessing (1969) writes of the necessity to find healing in the totally natural and irrational when a culture has, like ours, become so rational and "in control" that it is in fact insane. Martha, the novel's protagonist, spends quite a lot of time in the basement of the house where she lives, talking with Lynda, a woman well acquainted with mental hospitals from the inside:

> They called it "working." They might sit all night alone in Lynda's living room hardly saying a word, yet listening, trying to be receptive, to be alert. An idea might come out of it; or perhaps not. Or they might sound out this or that word, or phrase, or thought, by letting it lie on the air where they could get a sense of it, a feel, a taste; so that it might accumulate other sounds, words, ideas, like it. Sometimes they talked, trying not to talk too rationally or logically, merely letting talk flow, since in the spaces between words, sentences, something else might come in. They did not really know what they were doing, or how, really, they did it. Yet out of all this material gathered, they began to get glimpses of a new sort of understanding.
>
> They had no word for that either. Talking about it, or around it, they tended to slip back into talking about Lynda's being mad.
>
> Perhaps it was because if society is so organized, or rather has so grown, that it will not admit what one knows to be true, will not admit it, that is, except as it comes out perverted, through madness, then it is through madness and its variants it must be sought after.
>
> An essential fact was that if Lynda had not been mad, had not tested certain limits, then some of the things they discovered would have frightened them so badly they would not have been able to go on. (pp. 374-375)

The evening of January 9, Sarah took all the pictures in her house off the walls, "to avoid breakage," she said. At about 5:30 the next morning an earthquake shook Seal Harbor. The earth stabilized a little sooner than Sarah did, but not much. On January 14 she came to my house for a therapy session, wearing a jaunty hat, purchased a few minutes before. With a mischievous smile she explained that it was her "halfway hat."

During that session she became quite agitated and revealed that a woman had refused to go on a trip with her and Sam because of Sarah's "mental condition." We talked about the reality that a lot of people do feel that way. She had met such attitudes many times before, but the quality of her experience during this episode had left her open, unprepared to meet those who could relate to her only in socially negative terms. I realized that, true to her new hat, our work was only half finished. Sarah had found a better connection to herself, but she had still to find her place in the community.

Colette, who had been with Sarah during the darkest nights of psychosis, suggested we all meet together. She pointed out that everyone, not only Sarah, needed a ritual in order to be comfortable with each other in the world of everyday reality. A few days later, Mary, another friend, dreamed that we all got together and had a party to celebrate Sarah's successful passage.

It sounded like a good idea in theory, but whenever I imagined actually doing something of the sort I felt embarrassed. It was all very well to deal with these things so unconventionally while Sarah was mad, but *now* . . .? The inner David threatened to engulf me. I struggled with the unspoken question for several days before accepting that I had gone too far along my path to leave it now. To fail to honor the images Colette and Mary had given me would violate everything we had achieved.

In the meantime Sarah made a blackberry pie. On January 19 she celebrated her mother's birthday for the first time ever. Then she wrote:

> Here, use these large buttons
> Ones from my mom's coat
> We will make a blueberry pie
> And celebrate her 60th birthday
> I've celebrated none
> For Margaret Elizabeth Smith
> Born six decades ago
> Killed when I was six
>
> I wanted her to know
> That I care and that
> She was so special
> With a kindness that could
> Never be replaced

It was my mother's death
That sustained me not
My father's life or his
Future wife

Mother's death a
Harsh blow to little hearts
Of golden glow

The following weekend, on January 27, Sarah, Sam, Katy, and 15
friends joined me in a ritual followed by a potluck dinner. Winter Wolf,
a contemporary tribal drummer, gave forth the native heartbeat of the
earth until everyone had arrived. Then I put on a ceremonial robe and
spoke as follows:

Colette imagined and Mary dreamed that we gathered together
to make sacred the event in which we have all participated, to
acknowledge and celebrate our mutual bond. We have come here
today to do it. Sarah Petrovici crossed over into another world, the
world of pure spirit. Now she has returned, successfully and safely,
to the world of ordinary reality. She went to find the mother who
was murdered when Sarah was a small child. She came back with
a new name that was given her there, a secret name to hold in her
heart. She came back with poems and with ideas for new paintings.
She gave birth to herself and will be with us here in a new way, a
part of this community as she has never been before.

Sarah, we rejoice with you for your safe passage, and welcome
you into your new life here. You made your journey for all of us,
not for yourself alone, and each of us has been with you during a
part of it. Recognizing the importance of what you have done for
us, Rose has made you a pin, silver with lapis and a sliver of moon-
stone. Wear it proudly as a sign of your passage. Silver and moon-
stone hint at the feminine nature of your crossing. The circle of lapis
signifies the enduring wholeness you can achieve if you complete
your sacred task. For yourself, and for us, you have been called to
build a bridge to the other world, a bridge of poems, paintings, and
tellings of what you have learned, what you have seen and experienced. You are asked to heal a painful separation between this world
and the world of spirit. We all share this profound wound with you.
Almost all contemporary Western men and women participate in a
split between everyday life and the life of the spirit.

The traditions, even the language of Western medicine are harsh
and unconnected to the reality of what we who are here today have
experienced. Driven by fear and ignorance, traditional medicine and
psychology call people like Sarah schizophrenic, crazy, insane, thereby justifying shutting them up in hospitals, cutting them and the rest
of us off from the healing process that the psyche is trying to accomplish. Sarah pointed out to me the other day that schizophrenics
don't get colds; and I told her about the fact that schizophrenics
don't get cancer. Colds and cancer are the two primary diseases of

this time and place. Both can be cured by schizophrenia! Think about that.

The psyche knows how to heal itself. In passages like Sarah's, what we have to do is pay attention and take seriously the processes the psyche initiates, the language and images it gives us. Other times and places have been more connected to the realities of psyche and spirit that Sarah has experienced and the rest of us have experienced through her. Ancient religious mysteries, contemporary religious mysticism, and so-called primitive people know about death and rebirth, the dark night of the soul, transformation, vision quest, shamanistic initiation. These are the ways, the languages and images of spiritual reality, that inform psyche's self-healing.

Sometimes a transformation process is long, slow, and undramatic. Sarah's has been sudden and dramatic. Throughout her experience she spoke frequently in images of nuclear energy. It is as if a nuclear explosion took place in her psyche. One thing we all felt was the enormous amount of energy that was released, physical energy transformed abruptly into spiritual energy, body becoming psyche. We all worried about when Sarah—and therefore all of us—would begin to get some sleep. But so much energy had become available to her that she didn't need to sleep. Some of us heard Sarah say she had become contaminated by the radiation that had been released. Those of us who insisted on touching her anyway, who agreed to enter into this process with her, have in fact taken on some psychological radiation. We have experienced it in various ways, some positive, some negative.

We all know that nuclear energy can be used either destructively or creatively. All of us here need to find creative and constructive use for what we have been through together so we will not be hurt by it. For better or worse, the Age of Aquarius is also the nuclear age, and we are the people who must find ways to live together and work together to carry the power of the psyche, the power of experiences like Sarah's, instead of washing our hands, isolating ourselves, and sending our scapegoats out alone into the wilderness as generations before us have done.

I have been deeply moved by the spirit of love and community that has come forth from all of you. Several of you have told me that your participation in Sarah's crossing has been extremely important. I'm going to stop talking now and hope that anyone who feels comfortable doing it will tell Sarah and the rest of us what the experience has meant to you.

Almost everyone spoke. Some even read poems they had written and others showed pictures they had painted. Before we ate together, Sarah spoke too, and read a poem that came to her while she was in the other world:

JOURNEY HALF WAY

Half way point on the journey into
The dark side of the soul
Each person retains the last breath bubble
Transferring love and life one to another

Ra's chamber opens
Geometric door
Pyramid luminosity overhead
Who dares open this passage after the
Two thousand year seal?

Luminosity of being in the dark side of the soul
Carrying, carrying, carrying
Quietly on padded feet
Upward tromp, tromp, tromp

A downward slide on the matrix of life
To a thunk of deafening solitude
And isolation for an undetermined time

A shaft of light
Cut across a room
Child's play for the imagination
Carries thought

Remember
Correct the language
Allow the mind to be free
Correct the thought
Set the mind free
Oh little brave soul around the mountain
Soar to be free
Eagle flap, flap into the night

This has been Sarah's story, but also my own. The Redman knows that in telling and listening to our personal stories we become connected to a larger tale, one that the spirits are trying to bring forth into the world. Alone, each of us receives a small piece of the story, a piece essential to the whole. By telling, and listening, and putting together the fragments we hear, we begin to get inklings of something larger. When we can live in conscious relation to and acceptance of the whole story, then personal matters will find their proper perspective and we will be able to live with one another. When that day comes, I imagine analysts will be obsolete and we will all know how to serve the healing function in each other, as a natural and integral part of life.

But that is far in the future. Now it is February. Next month, around the time of the equinox, the spirits will go back to the underworld and the tourists return to Seal Harbor.

REFERENCES

Cameron, A. (1981). *Daughters of copper woman.* Vancouver, BC: Press Gang Publishers.
Holm, B. (1972). *Crooked beak of heaven.* Seattle: University of Washington Press.
Jung, C. G. (1961). *Memories, dreams, reflections.* New York: Pantheon.
Lessing, D. (1969). *The four-gated city.* New York: Bantam Books.
Perry, J. W. (1974). *The far side of madness.* Englewood Cliffs, NJ: Prentice-Hall.

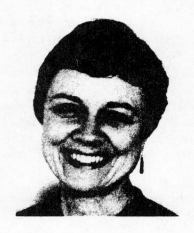

Marilyn Nagy

The *Lumen Naturae:*
Soul of the Psychotherapeutic Relationship

Marilyn Nagy is a Jungian analyst living and practicing in Palo Alto, where she is a professional member of the C. G. Jung Institute of San Francisco. She trained at the Jung Institute in Zurich and practiced for many years in Switzerland, where her two children were also born. Since returning to the United States in 1975 her time has been given to family, practice, and cross-disciplinary study in philosophy. A dissertation/book on Jung's philosophy is in its final stages.

945 Middlefield Road
Palo Alto, California 94301

One of the great heroes of Jung's later years was an irascible and passionate physician who was always being hounded out of town by his professional colleagues but was sought out and loved by his patients. Theophrastus Bombast von Hohenheim—known to us as the Renaissance physician and alchemist Paracelsus—grew up in the Swiss town of Einsiedeln, in the shadow of the famous Benedictine abbey which had been a pilgrimage center already for hundreds of years. Paracelsus combined in his person two very typically Swiss characteristics: an attitude of inner piety and a fierce independence of thinking. He remained his whole life long a devoted "son of the church" but in his work and in his writing he made such revolutionary changes in how medicine was understood and practiced that many people doubted both his faith and his sanity.

Paracelsus succeeded as quite a young man in making a spectacular cure of a prominent citizen of Basel, and, partly as a result of this cure, he was named official town physician of the city of Basel, a post which promised prestige and security. But he despised the customs of the town, lectured at the university in German instead of in Latin, and boasted of his achievements in such an unconscionable manner that his colleagues took the next opportunity to betray him and he was soon driven out of town. The rest of his life was spent as a wandering physician, mostly in the cities and armies of Austria, Germany, and Switzerland, though he also seems to have traveled as far as Spain, England, and even Sweden. He was never more than a year in one place, and often just a few weeks or even days, for he neither would nor could keep from dissentious and innovative behavior. As a medical doctor he insisted on performing surgery as well, which in those days was lowly barber's or army field surgeon's work. He made chemical analyses of the waters of famous spas, did urinalysis, insisted on antisepsis of wounds, and prescribed laudanum (probably opium) for pain. Worst of all, however, was what he wrote in his many books about the causes and cure of illness, for he violently disagreed with the theories that had been taught for hundreds of years in medical faculties at the universities.

What Paracelsus rejected were ancient Greek and scholastic views that reduced illness to a humoral disorder in the material elements of the body: to its earth, its air, its fire, or its water. That will not do at all, said Paracelsus. The only way to learn about illness and about the human being is through *direct, personal experience*. You must read nature's book with your feet, he wrote (Hall, 1969). That meant getting away from rationalized theories:

> It is not title and eloquence, nor the knowledge of languages, nor the reading of many books, however ornamental, that are the requirements of a physician, but the deepest knowledge of things themselves and of nature's secrets, and this knowledge outweighs all else. (Paracelsus, 1942/1951)

One must be with real people in the world, listening to a story of a strange cure told at a wayside inn, observing not only the pathology but also the life circumstances of an ill woman, not despising the wisdom of the gypsies, studying what actually happens in the chemical retort as it is held over the fire.

But *experience* also meant much more, for Paracelsus. He was not really an empiricist in our present-day sense of that term. What is of primary importance, he thought, is that we experience and understand how nature operates *in ourselves*. There is an *ens seminis*—a seminal essence, or an *Archeus*—a spiritual principle, which gives form and substance to each one of the objects of nature and determines the course of its existence. The spirit pervades the whole of the universe, so that each individual thing has its own proper qualities. But the spirit of each individual thing also shares in the cosmic spirit which informs the universe *as object*. Since human beings are the last and highest of God's creation (and here Paracelsus is a faithful medieval Christian) they have within their own natures something of the spirit of every other part of nature. This is the ancient doctrine of the microcosm and the macrocosm, combined with the even more ancient idea of a hierarchy of being. It means: As it is with me, so is it in the universe. Obversely: As it is in nature as a whole, so is it within my own soul. Further: There is an element inside me (the naturalist or the physician) which corresponds to the illness of this woman, or the properties of that plant (Pagel, 1958). So if I want to know what it is like, there is an "internal" path to knowledge that is more direct than the rational study of external objects. I must only come into sympathetic relationship with that *in me* which is identical with that *outside* me in order to know it truly. The knowledge obtained by this inner path is the *lumen naturae*—the light of nature. When I penetrate inside myself to that place of unity with the outer object, I "overhear" its inner mechanism and am thus enlightened.

Jung's (1944/1953a) interest in Paracelsus, and in the alchemical movement in which he was so important, stems largely from Paracelsus' doctrine of the *lumen naturae*. Four hundred years before the existence of psychology as a discipline that studies the workings of the human mind, Paracelsus' theory that we "know" by means of the sympathetic attractive force between like and like describes what we today undertsand as the *projective field*. Whatever qualities we have that are unknown to us we experience first of all in projection. Our capacity to experience beauty may become known to us only at the sight of a rose in bloom or upon hearing a concert. We know ourselves as never before when we fall in love. Many a young person discovers a fierce competitive soul only in the moment when someone else gets an A in the exam or wins at tennis. All these experiences of knowing depend on the fact that our *emotional responses* connect us to the outer world, and by reflection to the unconscious psychic world within us. The fact of projection is a crucial, if commonplace, fact of psychological work today. Jung was fascinated by Paracelsus and by the world of alchemy of which he was a part because the alchemists give us through their projective imagery an open window into the psychology of the Renaissance. Jung also thought that by understanding these ancient images and ideas he could better understand the dreams of modern people.

Whether or not Paracelsus' theory of the *lumen naturae*—of knowledge of the world through knowledge of myself—really applies to modern experience depends on whether we believe that trees and stones and earth and water are somehow alive as we are alive, and that we share a common quality with all other objects in such a way that we are bonded to each other. That is a matter for dispute; the issue will not soon be decided.

Where the doctrine of the *lumen naturae* does however indisputably apply is in the arena of *psychotherapeutic relationship*. This is the point I've been getting to, because it is here that Jung has made a unique contribution to our understanding of the healing factors in relationship. He was interested in the direct path in much the same way that Paracelsus was. Jung was entirely open to the factors of projection operating *between* the analyst and the client; he went so far as to invite them. In a classical Jungian analysis the patient does not lie on a couch with the analyst sitting invisibly behind the head of the couch. This was an analytical technique devised by Freud to encourage completely free association on the part of the patient and to ward off the possibility of countertransference projections on the part of the analyst by placing him or her in a higher, hidden, and supposedly more objective position in relationship to the patient. Jung taught instead that the analysand and the analyst are to sit across from one another in two similar chairs in a fully facing relationship. It is scarcely possible for there to be a more emotionally powerful constellation between human beings.

Even more than that, Jung said that the analyst's own countertransference feelings and fantasies about the analysand are important clues to what is going on. If there are none, it may even mean that nothing is going on in the therapy! How then is it possible to nevertheless provide for the patient a "safe container"—a therapeutic environment in which the patient feels that it is all right to explore to their depths the most disturbing emotions, without fear of being contaminated with contents that belong to the analyst's own psychic make-up? Who is to know what is your truth and what is mine, if both of us get involved in this thing?

The answer to this question is that, first, we can't avoid getting involved with one another even if we want not to. Secondly, if the analyst is not involved in some way, the relationship will never be believable and nothing therapeutic will occur. No real exchange of "knowing" will take place. Thirdly, it is absolutely crucial that the analyst must first have undergone a thorough personal analysis before attempting to offer therapy to others. The analyst must have gone along this path ahead of the patient. Jung (1944/1953b) was the first to insist that the personal analysis of the therapist is the primary requirement for entering the profession:

> If the analyst does not keep in touch with his unconscious objectively, there is no guarantee whatever that the patient will not fall into the unconscious of the analyst ... [The patient will] always find this vulnerable spot in the analyst, and he can be sure that, whenever something gets into him, it will be exactly in that place where he is without defence. That is the place where he is unconscious himself and where he is apt to make exactly the same projections as the patient. Then the condition of participation happens, ... a condition of personal contamination through mutual unconsciousness. (Par. 323)

With this proviso, that the therapist has already become conscious of the principal psychodynamic features of his or her own psychology and is continuing in a conscious personal developmental process, we may safely enter into the depths of the transformative relationship which is what analysis is. Knowing, and being known by another along the direct inner path of the *lumen naturae* is a unitive process of the highest order.

It is difficult to illustrate just how the acceptance and use of countertransference feelings enter into the analytic process without going into book-length detail on a particular case. Even so, the pertinent facts may escape us. I can perhaps offer a glimpse into the process by sharing two or three typical transference dreams which have come to me in recent years, and then say something about how I responded inwardly. What I would like to show is how the Jungian analyst needs self-knowledge both to make the connection with the analysand and also to keep separate the issues that are not pertinent to what is going on between them.

Dream 1

   Marilyn said that someday she would argue with me and get mad at me and then she showed me how she would do it. I thought that I might be pretty good at it myself. Then Marilyn started holding me as if I were a child. I liked it but I couldn't seem to relax completely. Somehow there was another woman there. She had white hair and might have been an analyst. She was helping the situation.

The dreamer has been through a psychotic break and emerged from it full of rage against the bad mother and weak father, which she had repressed for many years. We have already walked a long road together and there is a long road still to go. What does this dream about me getting mad at her mean? I have a painful (for me as a woman) reputation of calling the shots pretty much as they come in other parts of my life. Am I being reproached for being too harsh with the dreamer? But no, in fact I have followed her process with respect and attention. Again, I might be anxious that if there is too much confrontation she might not be able to stand it and our connection might be broken. Perhaps I am being warned to be careful not to do too much "analysis." That still doesn't "feel" right. Then I remember that confronting and dealing was just what the dreamer couldn't do with her mother. The next sentence in the dream says I am holding her as though she were a child. (That is something that I in fact never do, although I do sometimes hug a woman analysand on her way out the door.) Now I realize what the dreamer's unconscious psyche is saying. She is wanting in a symbolic sense to come into a mother-daughter relationship with me and to be raised up with none of that careful analytic deportment but with the instinctive sureness that a real mother has with her daughter. There will be a lot of quarreling but it won't mean our relationship is breaking up. It will mean that the connection is real and she can finally trust it. The white-haired analyst is the image of a "superior personality" who will oversee the process between us; it is something like a divine blessing. I feel completely reassured.

Dream 2

   I was at Marilyn's house. She was dressed in white, maybe a nurse's uniform. Then her husband came in. He was dressed casually, but had on a hat. He put on a video-tape of a piano concert and then got a phone call. He had to leave because he was a doctor and had to do surgery. Then I said, "Oh, by the way, I got laid off." I said

I had the same "on call" problem when I was in field service. Then I got into the back of a van. Marilyn was driving. I lit a cigarette but then put it out because I thought it might offend her.

I don't see clients in my home so the dreamer who comes to see me in my home is asking in a symbolic way for a more intimate relationship with me. The dreamer sees me as a nurse and my husband as a distinguished doctor and surgeon. I am in fact neither of these things and I have deeply ambivalent feelings about the authority role of the people "in white," perhaps especially so because I practice a profession so closely connected with medical tradition. The dreamer is talking with manly camaraderie with my "husband" about the problems men share when they are busy and always on call. Am I being set up for something? Is this a collusive trap? But no. The clue to the dream is the "Oh, by the way" sentence. The dreamer has been laid off from his job, something so painful that he cannot yet begin to face the full emotional impact of that fact. For the time being he absolutely needs me to be "clothed in white" with all the authority and protection of that role in order that the ego will not collapse. I don't much like the fact that he gets into the back of a van *I'm* driving, but the dream says it is to be a gentlemanly arrangement; he will douse his cigarette for my sake. I take that to mean that the dependency relationship between us will appear on the surface of our conscious relationship only in very subtle ways. It will be there, but we mustn't talk much about it.

Dream 3

I am with Marilyn. We have gone through a lot together. I express some need and she offers to hold me like a baby and give me a bottle. I'm really excited about this because she has never done that before. I say yes, and then I say no. I don't *really* want that.

In fact, the dreamer and I *have* been through a lot together. During much of that time the dreamer was overtly enraged at me because I refused to hold her. I had kept steady, but I couldn't help feeling great sorrow for the enormity of her need. I felt a lot of anger at her too; it's painful being on the receiving end of all that rage. The new thing in the dream, new for the dreamer and for me too, is the last sentence: "I don't *really* want that." I feel great relief. She does too. The boundaries will hold. We grin at each other.

REFERENCES

Hall, T. S. (1969). *Ideas of life and matter: Studies in the history of general physiology, 600 B.C.–1900 A.D.* (Vol. I). Chicago: The University of Chicago Press.

Jung, C. G. (1953a). Psychology and alchemy. In H. Read, M. Fordham, & G. Adler (Eds.) and R. Hull (Trans.), *The collected works of C. G. Jung* (Vol. 12). New York: Pantheon/Bollingen Series XX. (Original work published 1944).

Jung, C. G. (1953b). The symbolic life. In H. Read, M. Fordham, & G. Adler (Eds.) and R. Hull (Trans.), *The collected works of C. G. Jung* (Vol. 18). Princeton: Princeton University Press/Bollingen Series XX. (Original work published 1944).

Pagel, W. (1958). *Paracelsus: An introduction to philosophical medicine in the era of the Renaissance.* Basel, Switzerland: S. Karger.

Paracelsus: Selected writings (J. Jacobi, Ed.; N. Guterman, Trans.). (1951). Bollingen Series XXVIII. New York: Pantheon. (Original work published 1942.)

Paschal Bernard Baute

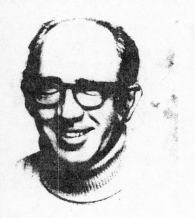

WHAT IF....
Religion and the Undiscovered Self

In his former life, Paschal was a Benedictine monk and priest (16 years). He has now been in private practice as a psychologist and marital therapist for 15 years. His doctoral project at the University of Pennsylvania was a phenomenological analysis of marital intimacy. Currently he is integrating behavioral, Jungian, spiritual, biblical, and faith perspectives in helping clients discover and love their shadows. He works in the rural Bluegrass country with his wife who is also a therapist. They have three children and one grandson. They publish materials for counselors and trainers.

6200 Winchester Road
Lexington, Kentucky 40509

See to it that the light in you is not darkness.
Luke 11:33

Once, out of time, the devil went for a walk with a friend. They saw a man ahead of them stoop down and pick up something from the ground.

"What did that man find?" asked the friend.

"A piece of truth," said the devil.

"Doesn't that disturb you?" asked the friend.

"No," said the devil, "I shall help him make a belief out of it. Before long, out of the vanity of his own discovery, he will end up worshipping his belief. Then he will become blind to all other truth!" And the devil laughed.

They walked further, and after a while the devil said: "I have even a better idea. These human creatures have such an intense need to worship, together with their need to reduce anything new to the acceptable familiar, I'll have the Jews believe that the Son of man is the Messiah, the Christ, and the Son of God!"

"What good will that do?" asked his friend.

"Don't you see?" said the devil, *"Worshipping him* blinds them to his Way: following the Light Source within in total response to God and to others. Since worship makes *him* the Source instead of owning it themselves, the result is that they keep on 'slaying' him and his message throughout time, all the while thinking they are giving glory to God!"

"I don't get it," said his friend.

"Well, it's making a vice out of necessity since his death did not 'do the trick.' By putting him up on the altar, they won't recognize how he transformed human consciousness and invited them to accept the Kingdom within. So these stupid humans remain passive Gospel-consumers (women more so), rather than becoming active and unique Gospel-creators!" And the devil roared with laughter.

"Wow!" said his friend, "that's really clever!"

"I haven't finished yet," said the devil, "I'll suggest so many concepts about God to make creeds and idols out of, that they'll end up slaying each other over who has the whole truth. His following will disintegrate into a thousand sects and cults, arguing and competing with one another like dogs over a bone. This will be such a scandal to nonbelievers that only fearful and lonely fools will want to become Christians. I'll promote the usage of belief to judge others and to feel secure—perversions of belief and secret forms of idolatry, which I craftily endorse!" And the devil snickered once more.

"Whew! said his friend, "I can't believe your cunning!"

"Neither can they," said the devil, "which is all to my benefit. But I'm never finished, I'll fill them with needing the safety of unquestioned beliefs and either having or hankering for many good things. Then they'll not be open to the strange better Way he lived and taught. Because responding would mean emptying their minds and hearts and *selves,* no one will be foolish or courageous enough to risk that." The devil cackled and crowed: "My slyness is so divine I am almost bursting! Last and best of all, humans will never realize that being so full of themselves is becoming just like me!" (Endless chortling . . .)

* * *

What if, finally:
—we don't need the devil to warp religion?
—most religion has been designed to escape from choosing by being chosen?
—we must "kill the Buddha on the road" to be free?
—all false images of God must be slain in order to release truly redemptive spiritual energy, and to allow the unknowable God to be God?
—the mind becomes one-pointed, and the "one point" is then removed?
—the radical transformation of human consciousness that Jesus lived and taught has not yet been apprehended?
—when we are full we are really empty, and only by emptying ourselves can we be filled?

Where do we go from the top of a 30-foot pole? (Zen saying)

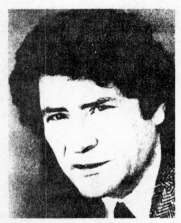

Michael Eigen

The Personal and Anonymous "I"

Michael Eigen is a psychologist who practices in Manhattan and lives in Brooklyn with his wife and son. He is author of *The Psychotic Self and Its Treatment* (New York: Jason Aronson) and co-editor of *Evil: Self and Culture* (New York: Human Sciences Press). He has published over 50 papers in professional journals. Michael Eigen is a senior member, control/training analyst, and on the faculty of the National Psychological Association for Psychoanalysis and also supervises and teaches at New Hope Guild and the Institute for Expressive Analysis (he has been associated with New Hope Guild for nearly 20 years). He gives bi-weekly seminars on Bion and Lacan. Some of the themes in the paper below are developed more fully in *The Psychotic Self and Its Treatment*.

225 Central Park West
New York, New York 10023

We all stand on the shoulders of the giants, Freud and Jung, and the basic structure of their thought is similar. They share an epistemology in which the unconscious is as unknowable as the physical universe, while, paradoxically, for both, the unconscious is the "true psychical reality." What is most basic about ourselves remains out of reach. We live through clues, hints, and convictions. But at times Jung felt he "knew" and perhaps Freud did also.

They share the conviction that psychic productions are inherently meaningful, including and especially the seemingly most random and mad events. Surface actions are read as messages concerning a deeper self. For both, "hallucinatory" structures follow innate timetables. Both emphasize the importance of megalomania in human life. Both stress polarities and the work of reversals. For both the story of each human being is crucial, yet something timeless and ahistorical marks human nature as well.

My focus here will be on a flaw in Jung's way of conceptualizing the personal and timeless in human nature. There is an important sense in which, I believe, his most basic terms are misleading and distort the self's journey. To see this clearly and in detail is all the more important inasmuch as Jung has such a grip on many of us. He has played such an important role in awakening, supporting, and furthering religious sensibility. He has helped give many of us courage to feel more deeply and to explore more thoroughly. He has extended the meaning of the term, "personal religion." And if, as Kathleen Raine (1982, pp. 267-298) observes, he confused the spiritual with the psychological, he has enabled us to better listen to the spirit and ourselves speak. Nevertheless, we must see through the trap.

Jung's Basic Terms

Jung's most basic polar terms are personal-collective, ego-self and complex-archetype. According to Jung, Freud's concern was with the personal unconscious and its complexes in relation to the ego. Jung affirms a deeper, numinous self as a primordial organizing structure, which he conceptualizes as an archetype of the collective unconscious. For Jung the ego is the center of consciousness, the world of time and space. The self is the center of the psychic totality and lays down the essential ground plan for the personality as a whole. The central drama is between these two main centers of subjectivity, ego and self: Will the individual realize, as best as possible, the basic game plan of the deeper self, or will he or she fall victim to the smaller ambitions of an ephemeral ego?

Ego and self may work creatively or destructively with each other. Jung usually blames the ego if things reach a destructive state of affairs, although he also celebrates the vast creative and destructive powers of the collective unconscious as such. Archetypal reality may have its way no matter what the ego does. Jung's usual script is that the ego is necessarily one-sided in its concern with everyday survival. Its focus becomes overly narrow and, in effect, tyrannical in its exclusion of those aspects of psychic life that do not fit in with its practical orientation. Jung romantically depicts the revenge the collective unconscious may wreak. The ego will be helpless against the storm its narrowness provokes. The collective unconscious tries to compensate for the ego's one-sided attitude. But if the ego cannot grow in consideration of greater psychic complexity, it courts disaster.

Too Great a Burden: The Warp that Runs through Our Beings

A certain snobbery runs through Jung's work. Jung speaks disparagingly of "mama's boys" and the personal weakness of neurotics. He recounts his own malingering in early adolescence and how he cured himself by sheer will and effort. He shouldered life's responsibilities, and a contempt for certain types of people who failed to do so never left him. This contempt for weakness constrasted dramatically with his empathy for psychically gifted individuals who may be psychotic. He could forgive a lot if the soul shone forth, if the individual could experience a genuine appreciation for the depths. As documented in the case of Sabina Spielrein, Jung (Carotenuto, 1984) could oscillate rapidly between disparagement and appreciation.

Jung appreciated a certain privileged position of the ego (as Freud did). Consciousness is our only medium of access to anything. We have intimations of our greater unconscious life through consciousness. He exhorted his weak charges to greater "moral" responsibility. The ego must take responsibility for its attitude; it must direct itself to other aspects of psychic reality; it must choose between alternative identifications and basic directions; it must not cave in in face of archetypal pressures; it must *meet* and elaborate but not give way to or merely fuse with deeper powers.

At the same time Jung revelled in the ego's undoing by powers beyond it. Like Freud, Jung loved the unconscious. He took pleasure in its triumphs. He enjoyed the ways it wounded the ego's narcissism. In this he was one with Freud, who envisioned psychoanalysis as a Copernican blow to the Western ego.

We meet a basic ambiguity or double ambivalence in Jung's thought. He honors the collective unconscious but notes that it is dangerous in its own right. He acknowledges the crucial role of consciousness but, with Freud, tends to treat the ego as a dangerous clown, one capable of poisoning the whole movement of psychic life. In mechanistic terms, he sees one system as exerting force on the other, reaction following action, as when the collective unconscious appears destructive in light of the ego's vanity.

It seems to me that Jung places too great a burden on the ego. He attributes too much of our misery to a narrow focus of consciousness. He seems to feel it is right and just if the unconscious reacts to the ego's smallness with hostility. He glories in descriptions of how the unconscious may, in certain instances, destroy one's whole personality in reaction to the ego's shortsightedness or tyrannical inflexibility. In the end the unconscious may prove to be a greater tyrant than the ego, but it is the ego that gets the blame. Jung is far more generous with the unconscious than with the ego.

I would hope that the deep unconscious were as generous. If the unconscious were so deep and vast as Jung imagines (for Jung it is synchronous with cosmic forces, expressive of the *Animus Mundi*), it could afford to respond to the narrow ego more empathically and reach out in more kindly ways. If the self is the greater power and more omniscient than the ego, surely it must possess resources to influence the latter without giving in to the need for wholesale destruction. Must the collective unconscious be a bully in order to get through to the ego? Isn't it big enough to know when such tactics work and when they are useless? If the self were a good-enough guide, if it truly had the interests of the psychic whole at heart, it would take into account the ego's wayward resistance and find a way to incorporate or work with it in the larger journey. In a profound sense, Jung's collective unconscious often mirrors rather than compensates the ego, and, at times, it is a horrific mirror indeed.

In a way Jung does not take far enough the notion that ego and self are cut from a common fabric. They are, after all, part of the *same* psyche, the *same* person. If, in the course of development, a person becomes warped, ego and self share in that warp. *The deep unconscious itself can become warped or ill* and not merely seem warped as a reflection of a distorted ego. This can happen as a result of the same processes that distort the ego.

In psychosis the very ground through which the ego emerges and needs support from undergoes deformation. The self may become destructive in response to a narrow ego, but the ego may be overly restrictive because of the warped foundation it is part of. In the latter instance, erstwhile ego fragments may resist the depths for good reason. Jungians refer to a weakness of the archetypal self in addition to a weakness or narrowness of the ego. The suggestion here is that the self is too weak to tolerate what it produces. This is much closer to the idea that in a pervasive psychic illness the self shares in the alterations undergone by the personality as a whole. The guiding function of the deeper self may go awry.

The collective unconscious does not stand totally uninfluenced by the individual's biography. How it works is part and parcel of the quality of a person's very being. The same basic intentionality or life script runs through the whole personality and characterizes ego and self, whatever the differences in role distribution. A warp in one's being affects collective unconscious and ego alike. One system is not to blame for the evil effects of the other. Both share and contribute to a common destiny.

Therapy sets the collective unconscious and not just the ego right. It addresses attitudes and themes that run through a person. In pathology, the deep unconscious, not just the ego, gets distorted. If a background screen is distorted, whatever appears on it automatically undergoes distortion. Therapy must slant in on the warp of a life and create a situation where the "background screen" rights itself. Jung's psychology can help do this but it also can exacerbate the warp. As Jung well knew, the deep unconscious itself must evolve but it will never be exempt from error and evil, not any more than the ego.

Jung shows how hard it is to follow the call of one's unfolding personality. But the difficulty lies deeper in our nature than the ego. The very structure of the self may be ill and discernment of spirits at every level may be called for. The overall movement of Jung's thought seems to be along the model of original innocence—maturational fall—sophisticated innocence or differentiated wholeness (Lowe, 1984). This model gets us off the hook prematurely, no matter how much we go through.

The interweaving of innocence and evil that runs through us is too thoroughgoing and complex to be divided up between psychic systems or parts of systems, or to be wished away by a vision of greater unity.

The Perversion of the Personal

Jung went off at the outset by making his primary dichotomy a collective and personal unconscious, thus foreclosing the personal at the deepest levels of psychic life. His psychology does not have any adequate concept which carries the full sense of what personal might mean. That he could misname Freud's unconscious "personal" is evidence of this, since Freud's unconscious is a kind of machine.

Freudian drives and ego functions can be anything but personal. Eros and Ananke are implacable forces and the psychopathic compromises the ego is driven to often suggest a collapse of the personal dimension in daily living. The mother or father who are objects of libidinal drives can scarcely be described simply or mainly in personal terms. The use of others as need-satisfying objects can become an addiction which competes with the development of one's true personal potential. Jung's calling Freud's psychology personal is perverse.

The complement of this is Jung's tendency to delete the personal from one's relationship to God. He emphasized the im- or transpersonal and used the term "personal" pejoratively. If a patient saw the therapist as God, Jung (1966) explained that the unconscious was "trying to *create* a god out of the person of the doctor . . . to free a vision of God from the veils of the personal" (p. 133). The overestimation of the therapist helped the patient develop "a transpersonal control-point . . . which allowed the psyche of the patient gradually to grow out of the pointless personal tie" (p. 135).

Jung did not fully develop the possibility that the patient was trying to open up or extend the meaning of the personal or that the patient turned to God to support a personal existence in face of parental failure to do so. There is much in one's relationship with God that is personal, and much in one's relationship to parents that is not. One's relationship to archetypal reality is often profoundly personal. In this regard, Jung too easily downplayed the Western experience of a personal God. He dangerously twisted and reduced the sense of the personal (Elkin, 1958, 1972).

The Personal and Anonymous I (or Self)

The perversion of the personal in Jung's work, nonetheless, helps to focus attention on an ambiguity inherent in self-experience. The relationship between Jung's self and ego focuses the dilemma with special intensity. Who is subject, who object—ego or self? For Jung each are both.

The ego is subject of consciousness, the self subject of the psyche as a whole. Self and ego are objects for one another yet each learns to respect the claims of the other as a subject to be reckoned with. Each feels wounded or helped by the intentions of the other and reacts accordingly.

Jung consistently describes the self as collective and transpersonal. Does a transpersonal subject say "I"? Is I-feeling part of the self? Is the self an I? Who calls the ego "it"? A divided ego? A greater I? A subject beyond I and you? Is the self anonymous or the most personal reality of all? The trail of the I vanishes into a deeper subject, the self, and beyond a leap through darkness, the I is Self, the Self I, yet more than I. When the Self opens up to the Unknowable Infinite, does the greatest Self of all say I (like Jahveh's "I am that I am")? And so on. *As far as we can trace, I and anonymity intertwine.*

No depth psychologist was more fascinated than Jung by the capacity of different aspects of the personality to behave as if they were autonomous centers of subjectivity. His image of psychic life was more an archipelago than flashlight. He saw the images thrown up by psychic life as sparks or "scintillae" given off by the unseeable fire of the World Soul.

Jung's sense of the intimacy yet otherness of the depths is shared by poets, philosophers, and mystics, and, increasingly, by psychologists. The past 200 years have seen a burgeoning of interest in I/not-I phenomena, the sense of the simultaneous distinction-union of self and other. Rimbaud's "I am an Other" and Whitman's "I am multitudes" are two of the many voices that resonate with Jung's concerns. Today, interest in the birth of the self is increasing momentum. Sectors of research are as intent upon decoding the originary self as the secrets of the physical universe (my book, *The Psychotic Self and Its Treatment* [Eigen, 1986], explores this and related themes in detail).

We cannot expect Jung to resolve the unresolvable. The problems latent in his simple polarization of ego and self plague more usual treatments of self as object of ego, as sum of social roles, as sum of id-super-ego-unconscious ego, and so on. At least Jung did not compromise his sense of self and ego as double subject-object, although we are left in a hall of mirrors. The more we learn, the more we appreciate the ways our sense of self and anonymity permeate our beings, yet leave room for something more.

REFERENCES

Carotenuto, A. (1984). *A secret symmetry.* New York: Pantheon.
Eigen, M. (1986). *The psychotic self and its treatment.* New York: Jason Aronson.
Elkin, H. (1958). On the origin of the self. *Psychoanalytic Review, 46,* 57-76.
Elkin, H. (1972). On selfhood and the development of ego structures in infancy. *Psychoanalytic Review, 59,* 389-416.

Jung, C. G. (1966). *Two essays on analytical psychology.* In H. Read, M. Fordham, & G. Adler (Eds.) and R. Hull (Trans.), *The collected works of C. G. Jung* (Vol. 7). Princeton: Princeton University Press/Bollingen Series XX.

Lowe, W. (1984). Innocence and experience: A theological exploration. In M. C. Nelson & M. Eigen (Eds.), *Evil: Self and Culture* (pp. 239-267). New York: Human Sciences Press.

Raine, K. (1982). *The human face of God.* New York: Thames & Hudson.

COMMENT

So, Trickster, up to your old familiar escapades again! I spend hours writing from my comfortable vantage point of an introverted-feeling-type an article on my personal relationship with the Divine Mother as my contribution to this issue of *VOICES,* and procrastinate about finding out the deadline. So our canny editors tell me my "comfortable" piece is too late—instead, say they, please respond to this paper (such a rich, provocative, extraverted-thinking-type paper), relying on your most inferior functions to judge, criticize, and reply in yesterday's mail on the wings of Mercury. By the balls of Hermes, how can I possibly do justice to Eigen's carefully thought-out essay, without even time to look at his references?!

One thing I have learned in dealing with Trickster: The longer one remains in the heroic attitude, the better Trickster likes it, and the more intense the game becomes. No, with Trickster one either has to out-trick him (I feel Trickster to be androgynous, but in this episode his masculinity seems predominant), quickly and completely to bring things to resolution, or play the fool so he loses interest. Of course there is a rare third: It's tricky, but it may get him to bend, to play with relatedness.

Eigen is right. This Dark Side of the Self extends its favors more equally to some than to others in ways that are truly unjust and unreasonable. Where is the balance and harmony in Trickster? Why else would a nice girl like me end up in a place like this? Why does Trickster always insist on playing with me when I am trying to be serious, mucking things up instead of making them right? I can't see the fairness to it either.

Come, Trickster Darling, be a lamb for once, instead of a fox, and help me with some of your intuitive brilliance instead of confusing things. Let us try together to see what Jung meant when he described Freud's theory as personalistic. Trained originally as a Freudian, I would have once looked for your, Trickster, origin in my relationship to my elder brothers, those shrewd ones before whom I was provoked to play the little clown. And I would have been right, as far as that goes. Jung has opened a window on your cosmic proportions, on your playing with me and them, complicating what could have been nice, straightforward brotherly love and twisting it into the bizarre, paradoxical nonsense that runs like a live wire through my most innocent relationships. Lord help me if I thought, as I once did, that I could catch you by analyzing my early brother-complexes; you will not be so easily pinned. Jung's way of seeing leads to changing the focus of the lens, beyond the history of one's lifetime into the timelessness of the archetypal world. *Of course,* Freud saw this aspect of the unconscious, but he chose a different lens because it was his task to get the factually oriented scientific minds of the time to see also. Jung took a leap that Freud could not afford to take, propelling his theory into the future in ways that currently supplement Freud—in a most convenient sense, a larger container has been given us.

Let's take you, Trickster, as another example. Looking at you, or rather, trying to catch a glimpse of you, I surely would agree with Eigen that the Self seems warped or even ill—at the very least, somewhat sadistic. But, these are ego-judgments. Who knows what havoc would be created by the pain of the profoundly wounded child with no recourse to the magic of your hermetic energy? You, who overcame the helplessness of infancy by thieving on a grand scale, are hard to fathom.

Michael Eigen, it would seem from ego's vantage point that few psychotics are healed by spontaneous compensatory functions of an inner healer. Perhaps you deal with this in your book, *The Psychotic Self and Its Treatment* which I have not seen. But the fact of mental illness does not negate the notion of the drive to wholeness. Since we cannot observe ourselves outside of our own families, much less outside of larger cultural influences, we cannot clearly know what balance is or even what wellness and illness would look like from another position. While therapy hopefully has some significant effect on the personal unconscious, I would say that it is not within our power as individuals to manipulate the collective unconscious, but to open ourselves to dialogue with more and more facts of the great unknown. To some this seems to represent all that is self-indulgent, a fatuous luxury; to others it is a matter of Life and Death. Analysis is serious play, as is worship. The prize of consciousness carries a high price at high risk. When the ego is not developed enough to take its side in the dialogue, other more developed egos tend to view it as tragic. We tend to see the weaknesses of others as tragic; you shrewdly picked up this tendency in Jung.

One of the ideas I looked at in my original essay which, thanks to Trickster, I arranged to have unpublished, is that many women come into the profession of psychotherapy in the role of midwives to the emergence of the feminine in the objective psyche (or collective unconscious), not, as is frequently supposed, because they are Fathers' daughters; their having gone through the patriarchal lateral labyrinths of medical and graduate schools does not change the fact that the basic movement toward healing is generated in many therapists from their wombs. It is not that women therapists are changing the objective psyche, but that they are present as witnesses and attendants to that process.

Michael Eigen, I strongly disagree with your statement that Jung was "foreclosing the personal at the deepest levels of conscious life." In showing us how Godliness is projected in the transference, Jung did see our striving to be related to parents and to God, but his achievement was to take us beyond the binds of childhood and into spiritual adulthood. While the God-energy is continuously incarnating in each individual, no one person can handle the role exclusively, though patients may hope that we can, and we therapists are susceptible to accepting their inflated perceptions. Jung and Freud were both exquisitely aware of the power of inflation provoked in the analyst by transferences, and insistent on analysts' needing to be analyzed. But I have never experienced Jung as you do, as having "downplayed the Western experience of a personal God." Jung insists that it is only through separation from the other than we can come into conscious relationship with it, and we cannot separate from that which we are absorbed by.

I believe that Jung, perhaps from behind a Trickster mask, is applauding your image of the intertwining "I and Anonymity," endless, vinelike, like the jen-tu energy paths of the Tao, and the Ida-Pingala of Hinduism.

I feel Trickster's eyes glistening as I begin to sound serious. Surely he will get me if I don't acknowledge him. Trickster, what would really be nice is if you could help me find a way to sneak in a little more from my original paper in a way that looks like it intended to be here, and not just having been tacked on because She wanted to be included. Perhaps sharing with Michael Eigen an example of my own personal effort to be with the Mother Goddess could accomplish three things: It could bring me into deeper relationship to Michael Eigen, it would bring Her in here where She wants to be, and it could be just the bit of inappropriate foolishness I need to get out of here. So, Michael Eigen, as a way of thanking you for your paper and your indulgence in my discussing it in a different style, I would like to give you something written during my early days of beginning to play seriously with Jung. In Zurich I first learned of the Schwarze Madonna, who is venerated in Einseideln, Switzerland, in the dark crypt beneath the magnificent cathedral at Chartres, and especially throughout Czechoslovakia. I was cared for as a child in New Orleans by both black and white mothers. She manifests Herself intensely to me in this form, and asked to be manifested to you:

SCHWARZE MADONNA

Black Mary, Black Mary, come down, come down!
In my cave I await you to speak in whispers
To sing, to sing, in smiling secrets
For we were born on the ebb-tide.
Black Mary, Mother, you understand
The journey in darkness, the black mist, crevice
The damp and deep pulsating caverns
Of those whose visions give birth to flame
Of those whose heat gives birth to vision.
Beneath the day, beyond the light,
In the southmost furnace of his red-rays, lingered
And with what strength you bore the thrill . . .
The throbbing power of his hot sword's-piercing;
O what bull's-might within you kept you
Whole, while soaring through that frenzy
Catapulted through night's spaces!
Nuit, Nuit! All is Nuit!
To those who choose the waning moon
To leap on in the spring to life . . .
Black Mary, I saw you, I saw you! You were
Dancing close with the Midnight Sun
You kissed in the sea, the night-tides high
You didn't even care who saw you
Knowing the warmth of the southwind's calling
I saw you reach for his full power
You took his All into your Nothing.
And when he found your velvet blackness lovely,
We cried for joy; then burned my candle brighter.

DELDON ANNE MCNEELY
816 Pershing Avenue
Lynchburg, Virginia 24503

Jean Houston

Pathos and Soul-Making

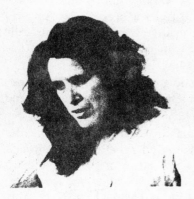

Jean Houston, Ph.D. is a pioneer in her work as a behavioral scientist emphasizing latent human capacities. She is the author or co-author (with her husband, Dr. Robert Masters, with whom she also co-directs The Foundation for Mind Research) of a number of books and numerous papers and articles. Her latest book, *Sacred Psychology*, a work on journeys of transformation, will be published in 1986.

Dr. Houston has taught on the faculties of Philosophy, Psychology, and Religion at Columbia University, Hunter College, The New School for Social Research, Marymount College, and the University of California. She was Visiting Distinguished Scholar of the University of Oklahoma and is Past-President of the Association for Humanistic Psychology. She has taught myth and sacred psychology on site in Egypt, Greece, India, and China. Dr. Houston is a much sought-after keynote speaker at conventions and other professional meetings. In 1985 she was elected Distinguished Educator of the Year by the National Teacher-Educator Association.

Box 3300
Pomona, New York 10970

> *Call the world, if you please,*
> *"The veil of Soul-making."*
> *Then you will find out*
> *the use of the world . . .*
>
> JOHN KEATS

Soul-making is not necessarily a happy thing. Critical parts of it are not. It almost always involves a painful excursion into pathos wherein the anguish is enormous and the suffering cracks the boundaries of what you thought you could bear. And yet the wounding pathos of your own human story may contain the seeds of healing and transformation in the larger mythic story which it reflects. As one notes in the Greek tragedy, the gods force themselves symptomatically into consciousness at the time of pathos. It is then that the protagonist grows into a larger sense of what life is all about. In times of pathos when one feels abandoned, perhaps even annihilated, there is occurring—at levels deeper than one's pain—the entry of the gods and the ennobling of the self. Thus, in high tragedy pathos is a divine process working in the human soul. How then can we build upon this ancient Hellenic insight and join a therapeutic process to a *therapeic* mode?

From the perspective of sacred psychology one would say that if you have a complex of some kind it probably began in pathos that was not

73

worked out to its source in the gods. That is why all complexes, at least in Jungian terms, have archetypal power. By working through the complex you find the gods within that are a challenge to a deeper life. Jung reminded us that "it is not a matter of indifference whether one calls something a 'mania' or a 'god.' To serve a mania is detestable and undignified, but to serve a god is full of meaning."

As seed-making begins with the wounding of the ovum by the sperm, soul-making begins with the wounding of the psyche, quite possibly by the gods.

Whether it be Krishna or Christ, Buddha, the great Goddess or the individuated Guides of one's own inner life, God may reach us through our affliction. Whether or not we are martyred, all of us get hurt, but we can be ennobled and extended by looking at this wounding in such a way that we move from the personal particular to the personal universal. This is the opposite of martyrdom. Is Oedipus martyred? Is Antigone martyred? Do they regard themselves as martyrs? Never. Consciousness in pathos is excruciatingly sensitized and has a vastly extended sensorium. Pathos has eyes and ears to see and hear what our normal eyes and ears cannot. What did Oedipus say at his moment of pathos, his mouth extended in great wailing: Aiiiiiiiiiiiiiiii!

Pathos opens the doors of our sensibility to a reality which remains closed to a normal point of view. When we feel our minds and our hearts breaking, this sometimes pushes us into a different topography, a different extension of reality. The pathos of Job extended him to the point that he touched the level of God and made even God feel guilty. And we suspect that as a result,

> The Lord blessed the latter end of Job more than his beginning: for he had fourteen thousand sheep, and six thousand camels, and a thousand yoke of oxen, and a thousand she-asses. He had also seven sons and three daughters.... After this lived Job an hundred and forty years, and saw his sons, and his sons' sons even four generations. (Job, 42:12, 13, 16)

In pathos Job became an archetype and had to be appropriately accoutred with the goods and services which accompany the archetypal life. A tragic-comic story, the tale of Job, but it tells a truth about what happens to us when we ground our pathos in the gods and allow the possibility of a mythic consummation. Not that you would want all those camels and she-asses....

In the cosmos of the psyche our lives may be under the governance of mythical categories. Now myths, as James Hillman has so brilliantly demonstrated, have their own patterns, systems, and symptomatologies. Critical to these is the fact that the pathos always happens in the myth.

Christ must have his crucifixion (there is even a school of thought that suggests that Christ arranged his own crucifixion.) Dionysus must be childish and attract Titanic enemies. Persephone must be carried down to the underworld and married to Darkness. Artemis must kill him who comes too close. Then there is the abundance of sacred wounding that marks the core of all great myths and their attending gods or heroes: Adam's rib, Achille's heel, Odin's eye, Orpheus' decapitation, Prometheus' liver, Zeus' split head, Pentheus' dismemberment, Job's boils, Jacob's broken hip, Isaiah's seared lips, Persephone's rape, Eros' burnt shoulder, Oedipus' eyes, Jesus' crucifixion. All of these myths of wounding carry with them the uncanny, the mysterious, the announcement that the sacred is entering into time. Each pre-figures a journey, a birth or re-birth, a turning point in the lives of gods and men. The possibility for *therapeia,* for healing and wholing, seems to require in sacred psychology the presence or happening of wounding. Wounding, of course, is always about the *breaking* or *penetration* or *opening* into the human flesh or spirit by a force or power or energy coming from beyond the ordinary recognized boundaries. In the journey of the psyche it is about the loss of boundaries of flesh or spirit that makes us vulnerable to be reached by large forces, large stories. Would there be much of a story around Jesus if he had been left to preach around Galilee and ply his trade as a carpenter and not been wounded unto death by the crucifixion, which paved the way for the resurrection? Instead of discrediting the phenomena of the myth as does a normative psychology, sacred psychology shows the ingeniousness and therapeutic power of myth in that it is able to illumine, save, and even redeem the sacrality of the phenomena around wounding that occurs in our lives. It is not that the *myth* is wrong, but rather that we are ignorant of its contents. Without the pathos of the myth there would be no wholeness to the larger story that the myth is always telling. Myth allows both hearer and teller to see the Pattern Which Connects. Similarly in our own existential times of wounding, pathos can tap us directly into the deeper topographical level of the psyche where we both reflect and join the Larger Story.

One of the most critical kinds of wounding that can happen accrues around issues of betrayal. Betrayal has always had an aweful and luminous quality surrounding it. It marks the end of primal trust, the terrible conditions which attend the taking of the next step. In all the great stories, scriptures, and myths it involves the loss of a simple and wholehearted faith in the Primal One, the bringer of justice, stability, and even love, whose word is binding, but binding within certain subtle conditions, the subtlety of which one is unable to fulfill. Consider these factors in the light of the two great myths of betrayal which dominate the Western mind. One is the myth of the Fall, wherein Adam and Eve are seen to have betrayed God, but could just as easily be seen to have been betrayed by their Creator. There they are, living as happy little mobile vegetables in Paradise. They have a naive and total faith in God, obey all His wishes, even the one concerning the Great Forbidden Act—the non-eating of the tree of distinctions. But then comes the snake who has all the lines, all the temptations, and carries the call to complexity. When Eve eats of the tree of the knowledge of distinctions, the trust is broken. But trust always has in it the seed of betrayal; the taboo implies and requires the transgression; the snake was in the garden from the beginning. God seems to have planned a big set-up. Eve's "betrayal" allows for the coming of reflection and therefore of consciousness. This may be why in the Judeo-Christian tradition there is so deep a fear of the feminine. The fear of the feminine is the fear of the coming of consciousness. And with consciousness you can transgress, transcend, deceive, evoke, evade, enter, and exit—in other words, *you can get somewhere,* instead of being stuck living on welfare in the Garden. Eve and Adam are thrust out of the Garden and are on their own. They have to begin living by their wits, using and growing their bodies and minds (establishing we can imagine many more dendritic networks in their brains) as they challenge their environment and struggle for survival. Meanwhile, back in Eden they have stopped boring God. Their conversation improves as does their pluck and cunning. They compound the distinctions even further, and in so doing create culture and civilization.

The second great Western myth of betrayal has to do with the coming of Christ. Things get so complex and out of hand in the world that God has to enter into human form in order to provide a new vision of meaning and possibility. But the key mystery of this story is not the Cross, it is the betrayal. James Hillman (1978, pp. 63-81) has a piece on betrayal in which he offers a fascinating discussion of what happens in the Christian story. To recapitulate his argument, Jesus is throughout the narrative in the New Testament very *sure* of his primal bonding with God the Father. "I and My Father are One," is his repeated assertion. Even throughout the week of the Passion, although he is a man of sorrows, his primal trust is not shaken. One can see it in his behavior before Pontius Pilate. He even asks forgiveness for his tormentors. But as the theme of betrayal unfolds its dark and mysterious course, it is raised to high ritual drama. It occurs in threes: by Judas, by the sleeping disciples, by Peter; and Peter's betrayal is repeated three times. This tells us that something high and holy is going on, and that betrayal is essential to the Christian Mystery. As Hillman has remarked,

> The sorrow at the supper, the agony in the garden, the cry on the cross seem repetitious of a same pattern, restatements of a same theme, each on a higher key, that a destiny is being realized, that a

transformation is being brought home to Jesus. In each of these betrayals he is forced to the terrible awareness of having been let down, failed, left alone. His love has been refused, his message mistaken, his call unattended, and his fate announced. (p. 69).

Then in the final moments when he is riveted to the Cross, denied and abandoned by everybody (although not by his mother and the other women), he feels the full human depth of the reality of the betrayal, and cries out the opening lines of the 22nd Psalm, the long lament about trust in God the Father:

> My God, My God, why hast thou forsaken me?

Hillman notes how the rest of the Psalm is significant for its images of betrayal by masculine powers:

> Why art thou so far from helping me, and from the words of my roaring? O my God, I cry in the daytime and thou answerest not; and in the night. . . . Yet thou art holy. . . . Our fathers trusted in thee; they trusted, and thou didst deliver them. . . . They trusted in thee, and were not confounded.

Then follow the early Judaic images of rescue by the Father from the forces of female generation:

> Thou art He that took me out of the womb: thou didst make me trust when I was upon my mother's breasts. I was cast upon thee from my birth: thou art my God from my mother's belly. Be not far from me; for trouble is near; for there is none to help. . . .

Then come the images of horror of being attacked by male animal powers:

> Many bulls have compassed me, strong bulls have beset me round. They open wide their mouth against me as a lion . . . the dogs have compassed me. The company of evil-doers have inclosed me: they pierced my hands and feet. . . .

Taken in full the Psalm reveals a poignant and powerful sense of betrayal by the Masculine Power. Hillman has cast a discerning eye on the fact of the narrative revealing a growing counterpoint of feminine or anima imagery to contrast with the imagery of masculine betrayal: Jesus washing the feet at the last supper (in the ancient Near East often a woman's function), the kiss of peace, the garden, the night, the cup, the barren woman on the way to Golgotha, the dream warning of Pilate's wife; the humiliation and weakness, and the women remaining at the cross after all but one of the men have fled. Finally, the finding of the risen Christ by the two Marys.

The implication here is that the man is born only when the feminine in him is released. The charismatic cocky miracle preacher is gone, and the full human is born. At the end of primal trust Jesus is available to the fullness of the human condition. He can die, gestate for three days, and be reborn. A fuller Love, a fuller beingness comes into existence.

This is also true of ourselves. Think throughout your life and note the holy and evolutionary qualities of betrayal. You will remember that trust and betrayal always contain each other. Therefore, it was the close relationships that more often than not carried the fullest agony of betrayal. It marks the expulsion from Eden into the empirical but evolutionary world of consciousness, growth, autonomy, and responsibility. It is only when we lose through betrayal our sense of intimate linkage with the other—be it mother or father or family or friend, or profession or ideology—and are thrust out into an unprotected existence, that we really begin to grow.

God grows by becoming human, and humans grow by "incorporating" the aspirations of God in themselves. The complete being, the possible human, as with Jesus, is the godly human, and the humanly god. As a result of the experience of betrayal in Paradise, we say "O felix culpa—O happy fall" which resulted in such a growth in reality. So for fuller life to begin, betrayal is necessary. The way to complexity and consciousness is through the crisis of betrayal, for it is then that you are provoked into extending and deepening your psyche in the world. In the wounding is the entry of the "gods," the entry of the More, insights and knowing that you could not assimilate before. The message of betrayal is always that things are much more than they seem.

Sadly, at the point of betrayal one can become calcified in the hard shell of alienation and unforgiveness, unable to love and given to one or another kind of sterile choice and distrustful fixation. In Hillman's discussion they could take a variety of forms: for example, revenge—an eye for an eye, a tooth for a tooth, a betrayal for a betrayal. Here a person can become so consumed with thoughts of revenge that he or she courts evil as a state of mind. All that you can say for revenge is that it may occasionally provide for some limited abreaction of emotion; otherwise it has the most abysmal shrinking effects upon consciousness. You cannot grow and be in a state of revenge. It is a pity that so many modern novels have revenge as their theme. Their constant reading can only have an insidious effect, as revenge gets reinforced as a thrilling and honorable form of behavior.

A second sterile choice is denial. If one has been let down in a relationship, one is tempted to deny the value altogether of the other person.

You see only their shadows, and many of their actions as prompted by demons. All previous idealizations reveal only their nether side in ugliness—mere compensations for darkness-driven behavior. There is a connection here with childhood innocence and ignorance, a failure to see the polarity and ambiguity inherent in everything. As such, it's a peculiarly Western form of distrust, for in the East the polarity of things is more often seen. From denial comes the continuous stream of judgments and evaluation which clutter up our perceivings of the other, the nonstop rule of consciousness by the Critic. With the Critic in residence relationship and resonance is denied; you cannot have these and have a constant commentary of evaluation going on. ("Let's talk about us . . . again.") Because the hope one had for the relationship has been compromised, the need for growing in mutuality with duration (always the mythical possibility in any close friendship—for as we all know, "they lived happily ever after") one comes to deny the possibility of love and relationship altogether. One's perspectives get warped and one stands out in ego consciousness from the primal unconscious trusting bond. Herein, one leaves the unconscious Garden of trust for self-conscious alienation in the world.

A third sterile choice is cynicism, which can also take the form of broken idealism. The most meaningful things in one's life are now seen as cheap and hollow frauds—the friendship, the church, the political cause, the profession—all pretense and fakery dedicated to setting you up for shooting you down. You'll stay on the ground from now on, thank you, with the dog *Cynis* chasing your own tail.

This leads to the ultimate sterility—self-betrayal. One betrays oneself in belittling one's deepest hope, value, ambition, story. The love letter that one wrote in the most exquisite feeling is dismissed as sentimental rubbish. The dream, the ambition is laughed away. It is the "nothing but" syndrome; one belittles one's deeps, and one becomes less in consequence. This finds its modern apotheosis in certain schools of analysis where one is encouraged to negatively justify oneself in terms of the meanest and most sordid actions. One is made to assume not the archetype of aspiration but the archetype of denigration. You are handed over to the enemy within and the nebbish has his day. People who are given to self-betrayal court the crash in themselves in others. Refusing to become what they can be, and cheating themselves with escapes and excuses, they often go into what Jung calls *uneigentlich leiden,* inauthentic suffering, whining and caviling, and boring the gods. Real suffering at least leads to wisdom and deepening. The suffering wrought through chronic addiction to one's own self-betrayal is merely erosive and uninteresting.

All of this leads of course to the supreme disease of betrayal—paranoia—wherein all human actions and affairs are seen under the rubric of betrayal as the constant of everything all of the time. This is surely the most dangerous disease in the world today, for the active practice of paranoia between great nations can lead to a combination of revenge, denial, cynicism, and self-betrayal that will involve the ultimate betrayal of Life itself. Paranoia is no longer a livable option.

The healing occurs in the revelation of the wider context. Often that means that the healing cannot happen for a long time, not until the context is larger, the Pattern that Connects is manifest. In the Christian mythos, one has to wait roughly 4,000 years (from the fortunate fall of Adam and Eve to the coming of Christ) for the redemption by God-forced-to-become-human, and the More to enter the world. This grows humankind, and, by inference, it also grows God. Meanwhile, in the struggle, ambiguity has been compounded, consciousness has grown, and culture and civilization have arisen. At last, everything is forgiven and reality looks deeper and more organic in the light of all the consequences. Meaning blooms.

The same is true with regard to our own betrayals. Time and forgiveness reveal how much the culture of the self has been extended by virtue of actions and reflections taken because of betrayal. They key issue here is forgiveness. Anybody can forgive a petty matter, but if one has been involved in a situation of deep trusting, of mutual flowing into each other, of rich coherence in which one has shared one's soul—and then is betrayed, then forgiveness takes on a momentous and evolutionary potency. This is the return to the Garden after the gaining of complexity. It is the willingness to enter into fully conscious partnership with the Creative Principle. It is the apotheosis of love, and the beginning of conscious and orchestral evolution, the life and work which you take up after your "resurrection."

This is why betrayal is such a strong theme in all the great religions and myths. It is the human gate to higher religious experience, it gives us the experience perhaps of God. In being betrayed the other becomes the instrument of God, bringing us to a tragedy which needs our ennoblement in order to arrive at understanding. And the only way to truly forgive is through love. This is the coming of the *Sophia,* the feminine wisdom principle in which love is restored to the event, love with the sense of necessity revealing the larger consequence and the deeper unfolding. Thus, for all its negativity, betrayal is an advance over primal trust for it leads to evolution and growth and the extension of the many qualities of love; it extends the universe in its challenges and vicissitudes, it grows the world and ourselves.

80

William Butler Yeats (1958) saw the promise of this world in "The Second Coming":

> Turning and turning in the widening gyre
> The falcon cannot hear the falconer;
> Things fall apart; the centre cannot hold;
> Mere anarchy is loosed upon the world,
> The blood-dimned tide is loosed, and everywhere
> The ceremony of innocence is drowned;
> The best lack all conviction, while the worst
> And what rough beast, its hour come 'round at last,
> Slouches towards Bethlehem to be born?

Who is this rough beast? Where does he lie within ourselves, this new post-Adamic beast who is at the same time the Holy Child trying to be born so that the world and self make sense again?

The point of our pathos is that it gives us the needed Fall to move beyond complacency into the high civilization of the psyche. It rips us from our moorings, destroys our world, and leaves us as rough beasts slouching toward goddedness and the renaissance of self and society.

And now for the terrible and unavoidable questions. Where and by whom were you wounded? What was the point of pathos in you? For therein you might find the gestations of your own possibility, the stigma that could well be the stigmata, the moment of your election into a larger reality. In the marking, in the wounding, a piece of the person has been struck by a god, drawn into the myth, and demanding from that a potent unfolding. The boar has wounded Ulysses' thigh. The angel of the crossing point has broken Jacob's hip. An apocryphal tradition speaks of Jesus having been crippled just before he began his ministry. The Fisher King who holds the secret to Grail Castle has a wound that will not heal.

Let us not cover up our holy wounds with band-aids. Let us find them, explore their larger dimensions, not for some paltry abreaction, but for the chance of realizing that we belong to a much wider order of things.

REFERENCES

Hillman, J. (1978). *Loose ends: Primary papers in archetypal psychology*. Dallas: Spring Publications.

Yeats, W. B. (1958). The second coming. In E. Sitwell (Ed.), *The Atlantic book of British and American poetry*. Boston: Little, Brown, & Co.

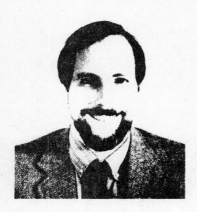

Phillip McGowan

Creativity and the Healing of the Soul

Phillip McGowan, J.D., M.A. is a candidate at the C. G. Jung Institute of Los Angeles and a member of the staff of the Hilda Kirsch Children's Center at the Institute. He is a psychotherapist in private practice with adults and children in Claremont, California, and in Los Angeles. A slightly modified version of this paper was presented to the C. G. Jung Club of Claremont on December 4, 1983.

301 Ashland #5
Santa Monica, California 90405

It is a well-documented fact that the Gods have become lost. Projections which in the past attached to stable religious images now inevitably arise on secular deities (Edinger, 1972). One such deity is creativity. It has the advantage of being an appropriate carrier of transpersonal contents, inasmuch as the creative process is unquestionably connected with the divine. However, a totally secular approach to creativity undermines the deeply religious nature of the process. It is not adequate to bring the ego into proper relationship with the archetypal source of the creative process. The emphasis on creativity and the creative process may be readily observed in the number of workshops, conferences, and lectures devoted to the theme. Even when creativity is not the main focus of the presentation, it may be attached to the main topic in a rather euphemistic manner, such as "creative divorce." This gives the impression that one can legitimize, or extract the guilt from one's actions by labeling them "creative." There is, of course, enough truth in this assertion to make it effective and appealing.

At a deeper level, however, creativity is inextricably bound to the process of analysis and to individuation in general. The experience of the creative process is the experience of the Self. Jung (1976) states this directly in *The Visions Seminars:*

> Only one who is confronted with an insoluble conflict knows something about the Self, and how the Self operates. Only in a situation where you are absolutely in need of a creative solution will you experience the source within yourself. Therefore any true analysis will lead you into a completely impossible situation where there is no answer, there is only a way to be created and you yourself cannot create it, but you depend upon the functioning of the creative sources within. (p. 457)

Here the word creative is used in the broadest sense and is equated with the solution of problems or conflicts. It is connected with the alchemical operation *solutio* in which ego rigidities are dissolved in the encounter with the Self (Edinger, 1985). Ordinarily, creativity is more frequently associated with the imagination and the imaginative, rather than its more general sense of "to cause to exist or to bring into being" (*American Heritage Dictionary,* 1978, p. 311). It is this link with the image which reveals its psychological importance. Images are the fundamental facts of psychology. In general, we might postulate two approaches to images: the scientific, and the aesthetic. The former forms the basis for analytical psychology as a science of images (Edinger, 1978). The latter is connected with art, art history, and aesthetics. However, such a distinction is by no means a settled affair, and is the subject of continuing debate.

Marie-Louise von Franz (1980) states the proposition in another way:

> Nothing in the human psyche is more destructive than unrealized, unconscious creative impulses. That is why a psychosis can, as a rule, be cured only if the patient can begin some creative activity, some creative shaping of the contents that are disturbing him. (p. 106)

I have chosen to examine the Chinese legend, *The Magic Brush* (Goodman & Spicer, 1974). It should be noted at the outset that no attempt will be made to discuss the relevance of the tale to Chinese culture. I have no real knowledge of Chinese culture and am only superficially acquainted with some of its products. Neither is it suggested that this is the most complete, nor the best vehicle for an examination of the creative process. However, *The Magic Brush* is useful because it is a story, the major theme of which is *transformation through the creative process alone.* The legend is as follows:

> Long ago in China there ruled a greedy Emperor. His treasures and lands were beyond counting—but always he wanted more. Under him, even the rich became poorer. And for the poor, each day was a new struggle to stay alive.
>
> In one small village, there lived a poor boy named Ma Lien. Every day he trudged off to gather firewood for the few coins he needed for food. He had no family, no friends, no time for play. He had only his dream to become a painter of pictures. Rich boys on their way to the village art school made fun of Ma Lien. "Poor boys can't go to school," they taunted. How Ma Lien envied them. To learn to put what their eyes saw into colors, shapes—into brush strokes on fine paper—that was Ma Lien's dream.
>
> Whenever he could, Ma Lien would climb into a tree to watch the teacher give the rich boys their art lessons. One day he was dis-

covered. "The beggar boy! He spies on us!" Ma Lien jumped from the tree and ran, but the art teacher caught him. "You are a thief!" shouted the teacher. "Trying to learn without paying is as bad as stealing!" And he beat on Ma Lien's head with a string of coins. "Painting is not for a poor boy like you! Go! Get to your wood gathering!" Sadly, Ma Lien went on his way. "How could he learn to paint if no one would teach him?" That evening, after his supper of plain rice and tea, Ma Lien sat watching the neighbor's chickens. In his mind, he drew each detail of feather and spur and beak. "No!" thought Ma Lien. "I will not give up my dream. I can be a painter of pictures."

The next day, pausing at a forest pool, Ma Lien was overwhelmed by the beauty of what he saw. "I must draw it!" cried Ma Lien. And so, with a twig for his brush and a smooth patch of dust, Ma Lien set to work. He forgot his wood gathering, forgot hunger, forgot time. He practiced drawing everything he knew.

Day after day Ma Lien would practice. One day, while resting, he fell fast asleep. In his sleep he dreamed that an old man came and spoke to him. "You have worked hard, Ma Lien, to make your dream come true. Here is a magic brush that will help you paint whatever you wish. But remember, use it only for the good of the people!" And with these words, the old man disappeared. When Ma Lien awoke, a golden brush was in his hand. Ma Lien raced home. "A brush! My own brush!" This day, he traded his firewood not for food, but for paper and a cake of ink. At the mountain pool, Ma Lien had learned with his eyes and heart every motion and fin and scale of the fish there. "I will paint a fish with my magic brush," thought Ma Lien. As he finished the tail, the fish suddenly leaped from the paper into a nearby water jug. "It is indeed a magic brush," gasped Ma Lien. "With my last stroke the fish has come to life!" Ma Lien remembered that in his dream the old man had instructed him to use the magic brush for the good of the people. "I will, I will!" vowed Ma Lien.

For the people of his village, Ma Lien magically painted into life buffalo to plow the fields and water wheels to irrigate them. These he freely gave to those in need. The villagers were overjoyed with their good fortune. Everyone prospered. Ma Lien was happy. One day in the marketplace, Ma Lien painted a giant crane. The villagers were so fascinated they failed to notice one of the Emperor's soldiers among them. As Ma Lien added the final brush stroke, the crane rose from the paper and flapped noisily into the air. Astounded, the soldier raced to tell the Emperor what he had seen.

Soon the Emperor's men arrived with the order to bring Ma Lien and his magic brush to the royal court. It was a long road from the village to the Imperial City of Peking. "Ma Lien!" greeted the Emperor. "We have heard of your great power. Now you will have the honor of painting for your Emperor. All my life I have wanted to see a real dragon breathing fire and smoke. All my life I have wanted to see a real phoenix. Paint them for me with your magic brush!" Ma Lien did not like the greedy Emperor. And so, instead of a phoenix and dragon, he painted an ugly cock and a huge toad. On his last brush stroke, the cock flew up and pecked the Emperor. The ugly toad croaked and jumped about. The Emperor was furious. "To the dungeon with this impudent beggar boy!" he commanded. "Give me his magic brush. I shall paint what I please for myself." As if it knew the hand that held it, the brush would not work its magic for the Emperor. His painting of a golden mountain became falling rock. His golden dragon, a snake that tried to bite him. The greedy Emperor barely escaped with his life.

The Emperor was a determined man. He had Ma Lien released from the dungeon. "Paint for me and I shall make you rich. I shall give you my daughter, the princess, as your bride." "I paint only for the good of the people," said Ma Lien. "Then paint an ocean!" commanded the Emperor. "Yes, that is a good idea," answered Ma Lien. "I will paint an ocean, your Celestial Majesty." Ma Lien's brush created the white crest of waves breaking on a blue-green sea. The Emperor was pleased. "Excellent," he said, "Excellent! Now paint me a ship, Ma Lien. Paint me a ship as I would go for a ride on this beautiful ocean of yours!" With the magic brush, Ma Lien painted the most elegant royal ship the Emperor had ever seen. "Magnificent!" said the Emperor. "Now paint me an ocean breeze!" "You mean wind, your Majesty?" asked Ma Lien. "Yes, wind!" said the Emperor. Ma Lien obeyed. He painted a wind so strong and fierce that the Emperor and his ship were swept far out to sea, and never seen again.

And so it was that a new Emperor came to rule over China, an Emperor who was kind and compassionate and wise. The story of the magic brush was celebrated throughout the four corners of the Celestial Kingdom. And Ma Lien? He returned to his village and grew to manhood, a painter of pictures. His wealth was in treasures more real than gold and silver—family, friends, and the art that was his life.

The Magic Brush lends itself to analysis as a fairy tale, for it contains the motif of the renewal of the King, which is the subject of countless fairy tales, as Marie-Louise von Franz (1975) has conclusively demonstrated. There are many methods used in such fairy tales to restore the King, but here the task is completed through the deeds of an artist. The Emperor of The Magic Brush has the requisite attributes of the kingship archetype. His name means "commander," and the terms "celestial" and "majesty" clearly refer to the divine aspects of the ruler. Jung (1955/1963) states that the king is the carrier of a myth or a statement of the collective unconscious.

> The outwardly paraphenalia of kingship show this very clearly. The crown symbolizes his relation to the sun, sending forth its rays; his bejeweled mantle is the starry firmament; the orb is a replica of the world; the lofty throne exalts him above the crowd; the address "Majesty" approximates him to the gods . . . the psyche of the whole nation was the true and ultimate basis of kingship: it was self-evi-

dent that the king was the magical source of welfare and prosperity for the entire organic community of man, animal, and plant; from him flowed the life and prosperity of his subjects, the increase of the herds, and the fertility of the land. (p. 258)

This relationship is expressed directly in *The Magic Brush*. The prosperity of the land is affected by the Emperor's greedy and egocentric attitudes. Hence the Emperor as a symbol of the ruling principle is imbalanced—"out of Tao," if you will—and in need of correction. There is some emphasis here on the moral deficiencies of the greedy Emperor, but, seen from a greater perspective, he is an innocent victim in the ceaseless process of the birth and decay of the dominants of the collective unconscious. The word "dominants" is synonymous with the concept of a ruling principle, and is particularly relevant to the discussion of the creative process in general and artists in particular, as we shall see. Most importantly, the alienated condition of modern man is due to the loss of dominants. There are many beliefs and philosophies that individuals attempt to foist off on the masses as ruling principles, or dominants. These do not, in fact, have the depth and power of a true dominant, and therefore do not, for any length of time, coalesce an organic community. Creative individuals, however, may encounter these latent dominants in an encounter with the unconscious. In this regard the implications of *The Magic Brush* are twofold. First, *image-making is a political solution*. Secondly, *the contact with the dominants of the collective unconscious through individual introverted activity has a healing effect upon the collective*. The second is, of course, a corollary of the first.

These notions are far from being realized in the modern world. The Western individual is tied to objects and seeks external solutions exclusively. He or she cannot see that it is not the object, but the archetype which stands behind the object which is the driving force. The artist, on the other hand, seeks solutions in the unconscious.

And yet, as we have noted, this motif of the renewal of the king is readily available in the products of the unconscious of the West. A dramatic parallel may be found in an alchemical allegory resurrected by C. G. Jung (1955/1963). It is entitled the "Allegoria Merlini" (pp. 266-274). In this tale a king is preparing for battle. He asks for a drink, but consumes so much water that edema results and he is forced to undergo elaborate treatment at the hands of Egyptian and Alexandrian physicians. Jung notes that the king's thirst "is due to his boundless concupiscence and egotism" (p. 3), and that egotism "is a necessary attribute of consciousness and is also its specific sin" (p. 271). Hence this symbolism is reflected in the concept of the ego-Self axis (Edinger, 1972, pp. 3-7). This theory postulates a cyclical process of ego-Self attachment and detachment. In terms of our tale then, the barren state of the Kingdom at the outset parallels the individual state of alienation of the artist-to-be. The emergence of the Old Wise Man and the subsequent renewal of the king would correspond to ego-Self attachment.

So frequently does the renewal of the king require the assistance of the feminine principle in Western stories that we might inquire into the nature of the feminine principle in *The Magic Brush*. There is no female character in the legend, and we might be tempted to conclude that the feminine plays no influence. This is not wise, for in the East it is so obvious to everyone that the feminine is the container of all life that little emphasis is necessary. For example, the Zen Oxherding Pictures of Kaku-An depict an entire individuation process in which no woman appears. However, closer inspection reveals that the inspiration for the process of transformation is nature herself, and each image depicts natural phenomena that correspond to the inner state of the discipline (Spiegleman, 1983). So too, in *The Magic Brush,* the beauty of the forest pool is the impetus to the transformation. It captivates Ma Lien and crystallizes his decision to become an artist. It would seem that the whole process is contained within and supported by nature, and that, in fact, the feminine element is supraordinate.

Closely connected with the cycle of inflation and alienation which emanates from the ossification and renewal of the Self is the orphan archetype. We know that Ma Lien is an orphan. This image has been elucidated most thoroughly by Edward F. Edinger (1978) in his masterful discussion of *Moby-Dick*. Edinger states:

> To Isaac and Judeo-Christianity, Ishmael is the adversary, the opposing alternative which must be rejected and repressed. But to himself Ishmael is the rejected orphan who through no fault of his own has been cruelly cast out and condemned to wander beyond the pale. Ishmael is, therefore, the prototype of the alienated man, the outsider who feels he has no place in the nature of things. (p. 15)

What does the orphan condition of Ma Lien suggest about the creative process? To begin with, we might state that all creative individuals are orphans. This is so because contact with the collective unconscious creates an inevitable isolation from—and conflict with—the societal collective; or, as Eric Neumann (1974) refers to it, the cultural canon. This clash is demonstrated in *The Magic Brush* in two ways. The most obvious is in the conflict between Ma Lien and the Emperor. Ma Lien does not like the Emperor as the authority of the cultural canon, and he resists him and eventually overcomes him.

Another image of this conflict occurs when Ma Lien is struck over the head by a string of coins by the art teacher. What is alluded to here is the fact that any institution, no matter how unorthodox appearing, may, in reality, be a representative of the cultural canon. The art school is for those who have money, as opposed to those who have talent. Therefore it defeats itself. Even so, rejection by society for lack of money and prestige could be perceived by Ma Lien as the bitterest of blows. Yet this does not occur. Ma Lien's response is not one of discouragement, but enlightenment. The blow to the head administered by the art teacher has the effect of the sharp rap of the Zen master. Coins are symbolic of the Self. They are round, precious, and relatively enduring. Ma Lien's defeat is, therefore, at the hands of the Self. The implication is that true genius is always a completely original phenomenon which can never be supported by any collective enterprise—even art schools. Once this fact is realized, it opens the way to the experience of the uniqueness of the Self. Hence what follows is instructive. Ma Lien renews his resolve, and then forgets everything: time, money, hunger. At this moment he is gripped by the creative process, and thus loses all contact with the day-to-day world. To forget "everything" means, in this case, everything ordinary. Eric Neumann (1974) puts the issue this way: "The creative man is stigmatized by his failure to abandon the self's directives toward wholeness in order to adapt himself to the reality of the environment and its dominant values" (p. 185). The Self dictates the conflict with collective adaptation and drives the ego into creative work. It would seem that all of the conflicts in creative people that surround such issues as adaptation to the environment as opposed to working on creative ideas, creative blocks of all kinds, and similar "conflicts of duty" arise from this archetypal collision between the Self and the cultural canon. Therefore, the modern individual who states with conviction, "I want to be creative!" is simultaneously entangling himself or herself in an orphan condition. The two are inextricably linked and every creative person suffers from profound experiences of alienation.

The orphan condition of the artist is invariably reflected in his or her personal history (Rothenberg, 1983). We mean by this a very specific psychological process. Although Ma Lien has no parents, there are many modern individuals who do have living parents, and yet still feel like orphans. This is due to the fact that the parents of gifted individuals rarely are capable of providing a psychological structure for the developing child. Physical needs are met while the needs of the psyche—that is, the imagination itself—are ignored. This has the effect of directly exposing the child psyche to the numinous energies of the archetypes. It is an experience which cannot possibly be assimilated by the tender psyche and must be split off. At the same time, it causes a lesion through which the creative material flows (Edinger, 1978, p. 4). It would seem that there is a direct relationship between wounding, inferiority, and rejection; and creativity. If the psychological needs of the child were met sufficiently, there would be no doorway to the collective unconscious, and the individual would be more likely to find an adaptation to the environment.

Concomitant with the orphan condition is the experience of depression in the creative process. This is suggested in the legend by Ma Lien's withdrawal from society into nature and by the fact that he forgets time, hunger, nearly everything. While this does not suggest the extreme condition of the "wilderness," it does indicate the withdrawal of libido into oneself, and the fact of being cut off from the world. Esther Harding (1970), in a paper entitled, "The Value and Meaning of Depression," indicates that there are two major reasons for depression. It may be caused by setbacks in life, or by major blocks such as the death of loved ones, serious illness, business failures, and so forth. The second cause, however, is that libido has fallen into the unconscious because some content is demanding conscious attention. The feeling of the depression is similar in both cases, but in the latter there is the opportunity to free the lost libido through a creative act.

In the case of Ma Lien, we see that both processes are operating. The withdrawal of libido occurs after a bitter experience; a tremendous disappointment. In addition, however, there is the creative act of drawing on the earth. This produces the experience of the Self through the Old Wise Man, and more importantly, it releases a tremendous quantity of libido in the form of the magic brush. When depression strikes, it is precisely this contact with our own earth which releases new libido (Harding, 1970, p. 3). This may entail actually gardening, but the extraction of a new idea from the unconscious is a form of psychological gardening.

Alchemical imagery is a powerful reminder of the archetypal nature of the creative process and of the encounter between the ego and the collective unconscious. The depressive phase of the creative process is equivalent to the *nigredo* of alchemy. The *nigredo* is always associated with the color black, which is symbolic of the darkening of consciousness which results in the feeling of sterility, despair, and isolation that we have discussed. Therefore, the alchemist declares:

> O happy gate of blackness . . . which art the passage to this so glorious change. Study, therefore, whosoever appliest thyself to this Art, only to know this secret, for to know this is to know all, but to be ignorant of this is to be ignorant of all. For putrefaction precedes the generation of every new form into existence. (Edinger, 1985, p. 149)

This puts the matter quite starkly. Consciousness of the necessity of depression and decay preceding any significant psychological transformation is "to know all." As with all things which relate to the unconscious, each piece of the puzzle is at once a separate, discrete phenomenon—and the whole thing; that is, the Self. While the lesson is easy enough to understand in its abstract condition, the experience of creative depression is assiduously avoided. Each creative act requires the ego to submit to the Self. Hence egocentricity is broken down repeatedly. Creativity is usually equated with the ecstatic moment of the release of the flow of libido. Therefore, the depressive phase is treated with contempt. The alchemists would have us turn this around. The depressive phase is the secret, the acceptance of which is "to know all." Blackness is the gateway to the creative unconscious.

In *The Magic Brush* there is a moral injunction. Ma Lien is to use the brush only for the good of the people. This notion introduces the problem of identification with the creative process. This is a subtle issue that occurs because of the unavoidable mistake of thinking that we are responsible for the creative product. Since all creative urges are derived from the unconscious, it is obvious that the ego is important only in the sense that it redeems the trapped libido. The idea itself does not belong to the ego, and identification with the creative process has very negative effects. Nevertheless, it is almost impossible not to be caught by the creative contents that exert a powerful pull on the ego.

A negative identification occurs when the ego equates the creative process with material concerns. This might be called the utilitarian or materialistic fantasy. The ego says, in effect, "What good is there in doing creative work if I cannot make any money at it?" In other words, since there is no guarantee of financial reward the entire enterprise is declared useless. This attitude betrays a residual identification with the Self. The ego deems itself the arbiter of reality who can conjure away those things it determines distasteful. This attitude is tantamount to dismissing the psyche as useless and puts us at war with our souls. The ego is not prepared for the contents which push up from the unconscious, nor does it easily accept the fact that the work must be done simply because *it* wants to be done. It would seem that depression would be a rather strong motivation for the ego to engage in the work. However, as we all know, it is precisely when we are cornered like this that we resent it the most, because we are forced to admit that there is something that is larger than we are.

A positive identification occurs by virtue of possession of the magic brush. That is, the artist touches the divine creative power and attributes this power to his personal attributes. Therefore, there is the necessity of a moral pronouncement. Ma Lien is instructed to use the brush only for the good of the people. In other words, it is not a personal talent, but a transpersonal force with the power to do great harm or good. The Old Wise Man is stating, in effect, do not identify with your product, but give it away. We are rarely so altruistic. But how is it true that if one undertakes some creative act that they are performing a service for their fellow humans? Recalling that von Franz considers unexpressed creative contents to be the most destructive, the point is that they are destructive not only to the individual, but to those around as well. It is rather like being continuously out of Tao. Everyone who comes into contact with someone who is out of sorts, who is at odds with himself or herself, is also irritated to a certain extent. When we pay attention to creative material we are performing a psychic house-cleaning which has a beneficial effect on those around us. In this sense we have the opportunity to give to others by taking ourselves seriously. We need not say anything about this. In fact, it can be argued that by talking about it we may negate the effect. But it seems certain that by redeeming this libido trapped in the unconscious we are contributing our share to the collective at large because we have transformed this content and need no longer project it or repress it.

That the artist can be a servant of the people is made clear in a letter which Jung (1975) wrote to Herbert Read in September 1960:

> The great problem of our time is that we don't understand what is happening to the world. We are confronted with the darkness of our soul, the unconscious. It sends up its dark and unrecognizable urges. It hollows out and hacks up the shapes of our culture and its historical dominants. We have no dominants any more, they are in the future. Our values are shifting, everything loses its certainty, even *sanctissima causalitas* has descended from the throne of the axioma and has become a mere field of probability. Who is the awe-inspiring guest who knocks at our door portentously? Fear precedes him, showing that ultimate values already flow towards him. Our hitherto believed values decay accordingly and our only certainty is that the new world will be something different from what we were used to. If any of his urges show some inclination to incarnate in a known shape, the creative artist will not trust it. He will say: "Thou art not what thou sayest," and he will hollow them out and hack them up. That is where we are now. They have not yet learned to discriminate between their willful mind and the objective manifestations of the psyche. They have not yet learned to be objective with their own psyche, i.e., [to discriminate] between the thing which you do and the thing that happens to you. When somebody has a happy hunch, he thinks that *he* is clever, or that something which he does not know does not exist. We are still in a shockingly primitive state of mind, and this is the main reason why we cannot become objective in psychic matters. . . . It is the great dream which has always spoken through the artist as mouthpiece. All his love and passion [his "values"] flow towards the coming guest to proclaim his arrival. (pp. 590-591)

This letter is an amplification of *The Magic Brush*. Jung, as the Old Wise Man, is pleading with the artist to use the brush for the good of the people. It is an injunction not to identify with the creative process precisely because it is the vehicle of "guest," the newly formed dominant still awaiting birth.

The Old Wise Man in the tale may be seen as the daimon of Ma Lien. The word "daimon" comes from the Greek word *daimonal,* meaning divide, distribute, allot, or assign. It originally referred to what Marie-Louise von Franz (1980) refers to as a "momentarily perceptible divine activity such as a startled horse, a failure in work, illnesses, madness, terror in certain natural spots" (p. 108). In this sense even skills or talents constitute *daimonai.* Eventually, there arose the notion that the daimon was a person's constant companion, and as early as the 4th century b.c., sacrifices were made to a good daimon as the house spirit.

For Plato the word daimon was synonymous with *theos* or God. In a famous passage in the *Symposium,* Diotima tells Socrates, "Eros is a mighty Daimon, and is halfway between God and man." Socrates asks, "What powers have they then?" She replies, "They are the envoys and interpreters that ply between heaven and earth, flying upwards with our worship and our prayers, and descending with the heavenly answers and commandments, and since they are between the two estates they weld both sides together and merge them into one great whole" (cited in von Franz, 1980). In Roman times the Greek notion of the daimon was reflected in the *genius* or *juno,* to which every citizen offered sacrifices upon his or her birthday. Apuleius insisted that the genius was the guardian of one's welfare, and, through careful attention to him, would assist one in dangerous situations.

It is apparent in *The Magic Brush* that the Old Wise Man represents Ma Lien's genius. He appears at a time of great turmoil and distress. Further, because Ma Lien unhesitatingly follows the counsel of the Old Wise Man, he is blessed with a full life. We might note also that it is Ma Lien's fidelity to his genius which overturns the greedy Emperor.

An example of how the genius influences one's personal life is described by Jung (1965) in *Memories, Dreams, and Reflections:*

> A book of mine is always a matter of fate. There is something unpredictable about the process of writing, and I cannot prescribe for myself any predetermined course. Thus this "autobiography" is now taking a direction quite different from what I had imagined at the beginning. It has become a necessity for me to write down my early memories. If I neglect to do so for a single day, unpleasant physical symptoms immediately follow. As soon as I set to work they vanish and my head feels perfectly clear. (p. vi)

This statement should be seen as a testimony to the extraordinary sensitivity of the unconscious to creative work. Abandoning a creative project, even for a single day, may produce extremely unpleasant symptoms.

Finally, the legend is a moving example of the living reality of the creative process and of the psyche itself. Indeed, it is stated explicitly in *The Magic Brush* that whatever Ma Lien draws come to life. This is a wonderful parallel to the experience of active imagination. In a lecture given in England in 1935, Jung (1968) gave a fascinating example of this psychological reality (pp. 190-191). He was consulted by an artist who was incapable of comprehending what Jung meant by active imagination. The patient had to take the train to consult Jung, and in the station was a poster of the Alps. On one occasion, while still perplexed about Jung's notion of active imagination, the artist determined to attempt to have a fantasy about the poster. To that end he imagined that he was in the poster and began to walk in the meadow which was pictured there. He encountered a creature with pointed ears which caused him to dismiss the fantasy. But, on second thought, he wondered if perhaps the fantasy was real. So he repeated the process and once again the fantasy unfolded in exactly the same manner, pointed-eared creature and all. This experiment convinced the artist of the reality of the psyche, and from that moment on he was capable of using active imagination. We might say that, at that moment, the images in the poster came to life. Prior to that, they were inanimate. Thus, Ma Lien's life becomes a paradigm for all creative individuals. The urge to capture images is the first indication of the workings of the Self. If followed with the correct attitude, it is a path to the living psyche. This is the opportunity of all creative individuals—to descend into the unconscious and touch the living psyche.

REFERENCES

American heritage dictionary. (1978). Boston: Houghton Mifflin Co.

Edinger, E. F. (1972). *Ego and archetype.* New York: G. P. Putnam's Sons.

Edinger, E. F. (1978). *Melville's Moby-Dick: A Jungian commentary.* New York New Directions Books.

Edinger, E. F. (1985). *Anatomy of the psyche.* LaSalle, IL: Open Court.

Goodman, R. B., & Spicer, R. A. (1974). *The magic brush* (R. Tabrah, Ed.). Honolulu: Island Heritage.

Harding, E. (1970). The value and meaning of depression. New York: The Analytical Psychology Club of New York.

Jung, C. G. (1963). Mysterium coniunctionis. In H. Read, M. Fordham, & G. Adler (Eds.) and R. Hull (Trans.), *The collected works of C. G. Jung* (Vol. 14, pp. 258-381). New York: Pantheon/Bollingen Series XX. (Original work published 1955).

Jung, C. G. (1965). *Memories, dreams, reflections* (A. Jaffé, Trans.). New York: Random House.

Jung, C. G. (1968). *Analytical psychology, Its theory and practice.* New York: Random House. (Original work published 1935).

Jung, C. G. (1969). Spirit and life. In H. Read, M. Fordham, & G. Adler (Eds.) and R. Hull (Trans.), *The collected works of C. G. Jung* (Vol. 8, pp. 319-337). Princeton: Princeton University Press/Bollingen Series XX.

Jung, C. G. (1975). *Letters* (Vol. 2, G. Adler & A Jaffé, Eds.; R. Hull, Trans.) New York: Random House.

Jung, C. G. (1976). *The visions seminars.* New York: Spring Publications.

Neumann, E. (1974). *Art and the creative unconscious.* Princeton: Princeton University Press.

Rothenberg, R-E. (1983). The orphan archetype. *Psychological Perspectives, 14*(2), 181-194.

Spiegleman, J. M. (1983, Winter). *Analysis of the Zen oxherding pictures.* Seminar given at the C. G. Jung Institute of Los Angeles.

von Franz, M-L. (1975). *Interpretation of fairy tales.* New York: Spring Publications.

von Franz, M-L. (1980). *Projection and re-collection in Jungian psychology.* LaSalle, IL: Open Court.

John R. Haule

Soul-Loss and Restoration:
A Study in Countertransference

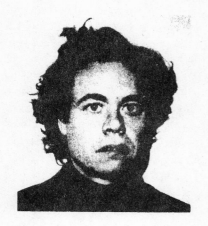

John R. Haule, Ph.D. (Religion), Temple University; diploma, C. G. Jung Institute-Zurich, is in private practice as a Jungian analyst. He was formerly assistant professor of philosophy and religion, Northeastern University (Boston). He is President of the New England Society of Jungian Analysts and member of the training board, C. G. Jung Institute–Boston. Dr. Haule has been published in *Journal of Analytical Psychology, Psychoanalytic Review, Religion, Journal of Religion and Health, Journal of Psychology and Theology, Dictionary of Pastoral Care and Counseling,* and elsewhere.

48 Chestnut Terrace
Newton Centre, Massachusetts 02159

The notion of *soul* is fundamental to Analytical Psychology. Sometimes Jung (1931/1960) uses *soul* interchangeably with *psyche*. More frequently, however, he uses it to refer to a subpersonality: a psychological content (a) with a certain measure of autonomy, (b) in which spontaneity is inherent, and (c) which is partially unconscious (Jung, 1921/ 1971, par. 419). Clearly this is not the theological formulation of Christianity, but rather a matter of human experience; something more like the conception found in preliterate societies (Jung, 1927/1964, par. 84). Phenomenologist of religion, Gerardus van der Leeuw (1933/1963) sees soul as fundamental for human self-understanding: "That man represents his soul by his own image implies . . . that in the soul man seeks to fathom his own essence, which is concealed from him [from his ego] and yet superior to him" (vol. 1, p. 286). Soul is therefore not merely subjective, as our western prejudice might incline us to suppose. "Soul phenomena," not at all reducible to consciousness, are "objectively real" (Jung, 1931/1960, par. 667): We can only very partially suppress our emotions and moods and cannot change them; our dreams cannot be controlled; we have ideas we cannot get out of our heads; our memory plays tricks on us; fantasies arise spontaneously; and neurotic symptoms humiliate us.

Understanding disease as loss of soul, either strayed away or stolen, is extremely widespread among the preliterate peoples of North and South America, and particularly (referring to the paradigm incident narrated below) in the Amazonian and Andean regions (Eliade, 1951/1964; p. 327; Hultkrantz, 1967, p. 131). It is also widespread in Africa, Australia,

Oceania, North Asia (Eliade, 1951/1964, p. 335) and India (Eliade, 1954/1969, pp. 312-317). In the Americas, it is generally believed that an individual has two types of soul: a bodily soul (or several) which grants life, movement, and consciousness to the body; and a dream-soul which wanders through the dream landscape while we sleep and can get lost or stolen (Hultkrantz, 1967, p. 131; Underhill, 1965, p. 63). The shaman can diagnose a very large array of ailments as due to soul-loss (Underhill, 1965, p. 89). The central symptoms, however, are a feeling of discouragement, lack of energy (Underhill, 1965, p. 89), unconsciousness, and mental disorders (Hultkrantz, 1967, pp. 89f). One feels listless, morose, unable to face the tasks of the day (Jung, 1939/1969, par. 213).

In preliterate societies, the shaman is the expert in matters of soul; "He alone 'sees' it, for he knows its 'form' and its destiny" (Eliade, 1951/1964, p. 8). Generally the shaman retrieves a lost soul by sending his or her own soul after it; that is, by attaining an altered state of consciousness or ecstasy in which his or her soul leaves its body and enters the landscape described in myth. Thus a shaman may be defined as a specialist "who can cross over into the supernatural world at will to deal with the forces that influence and even determine the events of waking life" (Harner, 1973, p. 16). The shaman heals, it may be said, by making the transcendent/mythic world real and relevant for everyday experience. "The myths ... can be reexperienced, ordered, intensified, given artistic shape and communicated by means of the trance of an individual specially prepared for this activity" (Nowak, 1977, p. 12).

In modern Western society, psychotherapists have become the experts in soul—at least as much as the clergy. I would like to discuss psychotherapy on the model of soul-loss and the restoration of soul. My fundamental assumptions, in agreement with Jung, are that preliterate societies know very well what they mean by loss of soul, namely a characteristic, potentially fatal depression; and that the shamanic finding and restoration of soul rely upon similarly distinctive kinds of experience, which may be located within the psychotherapeutic category we label transference/countertransference. In order to make this clear, I have organized my remarks around an instance of shamanic healing selected and condensed from anthropologist Florinda Donner's (1982) account of the year she spent living in every respect as a Yanomama Indian in the remote rain forests of the Amazon basin in Venezuela. What particularly recommends this narrative is that Donner herself became involved in the cure, thereby giving us the extraordinary chance to consider a traditional restoration of soul as experienced by an articulate Westerner (pp. 243-248).

Little four-year-old Texoma, eldest daughter of the polygynous family with which Donner lives, becomes listless and weepy while in the swamp on a frog-catching expedition. Donner carries her home, where she falls into a fitful sleep and develops a high temperature. The girl's mother has already been despondent for almost a week. Avoiding work and social contact, she has spent her time playing with the infant son of her co-wife, evidently preoccupied with her husband's absence on a raiding party to a tribe several days' journey distant. Presented with Texoma's illness, the mother is immediately convinced that the girl's soul has been lured away by a shaman of the enemy tribe. Donner denies this diagnosis, claiming that the child only has "the flu." She is so sure, she avers, that she can "feel it in my legs."

As this does not convince the mother, Donner fetches Texoma's great-uncle, Iramamowe, the community's most powerful shaman. He takes a dose of his hallucinogenic snuff and officially confirms that the soul is missing. In his trance, the shaman searches his visions carefully; but not being able to find the girl's soul, he calls in her playmates and Donner to help him search. Without the aid of drugs, they sweep with branches every inch of the community living space: eating and sleeping quarters, storage areas, pathways to the river, to the gardens, and to the latrine. Donner is told that she will "just know" if she finds the girl's soul. But these activities, too, prove fruitless. Convinced by the second day that an enemy shaman has stolen the girl's soul, Iramamowe is reduced to having to try to "suck" pathogens out of the girl's body via ritual sucking actions.

Donner finds herself "filled with an indescribable sense of help-lessness" at this turn of events and asks the shaman to command his spirit-helpers to assist her while she works a "water cure." Iramamowe questions her closely concerning her intentions and how they relate to the realities he knows. She reminds him that he has often said that he can see the spirits in her eyes and that his own spirit familiars "are already acquainted with me." She will be the sober instrument of the spirits while he will take the snuff and commune directly with them. As Iramamowe indicates his satisfaction with this arrangement, Donner organizes the women to bring her boiling water and the older boys to cut and heat palm fronds, as she employs her own grandmother's cure of "breaking the fever" with hot compresses. The struggle goes on all night long. At one point, Donner writes: "My assurance faltered. I mumbled a prayer for her with a fervor I had not had since I was a child. Looking up, I noticed Iramamowe gazing at me. He seemed anxious, as if aware of the mixture of feelings—magic, religion, and fear—fighting inside me. Determinedly, we went on chanting" (p. 247). At dawn the girl sits up and asks for water. Her fever is broken and her soul has returned. "Iramamowe stopped beside me on the way back to his hut. We did not talk, but I was certain we shared a moment of absolute understand-ing." (p. 248)

Before proceeding to analyze these events, the theme of my reading of the story can be summarized. I believe Donner has played an essential part in the healing, having found and restored the girl's soul; and she has done it by utilizing what psychotherapists will recognize as a class of countertransferential feelings.

Loss of Soul

There are two interpretations of the girl's illness. The Indians are convinced that her soul is lost, a matter of life and death. In our terms, she has lost her will to live, evidently because she feels like an abandoned child, her father likely dead and her mother despondent and no longer interested in her. It seems to be a matter of what might be called "sociosomatics," as formulated by Lévi-Strauss (1958/1967): "Physical integrity cannot withstand the dissolution of the social personality" (p. 161). The fact that family and community support have vanished, must leave her annihilated, a "nobody." The girl must be convinced that she has a reason to go on living, that she is loved, valued, and supported. This is a situation we encounter frequently with borderline and narcissistic patients whose powerful encounters with unconscious (archetypal) material have made them feel both "special" and isolated from humankind.

The diagnosis of soul-loss therefore requires that the symbolic foundations of community life be recovered, rehearsed, and reaffirmed.

Often our work consists primarily in helping people to discover the validity of their experience, and especially that others have had similar experiences.

On the other hand, Donner believes Texoma has a case of the flu. This is a trivial everyday diagnosis which says, in effect, "Don't worry, she'll be fine in a day or two." Superficially, there could indeed be a minor virus infection involved; but this does not necessarily deny the deeper reality to which the Yanomama are more sensitive than we. When Donner emphasizes her view of the illness by saying she can "feel it in my legs," I assume she believes herself to be imitating a Yanomama figure of speech. Consciously, she means only to reassure. However, in view of the fact that she actually does restore the girl's soul, she may be speaking more truly than she knows.

The Shaman's Trance

Universally, shamans perform their most important functions in an altered state of consciousness, achieved by fasting, dancing, drumming, meditation, and the like. In the northern portion of South America, potions and snuffs made from naturally growing narcotics are the most common means of attaining trance. Columbus himself was the first to report on the Indian's use of narcotic snuff (Reichel-Dolmatoff, 1975, p.

5). The trance is understood to bring about a "separation of soul" (Reichel-Dolmantoff, 1971, p. 174) or a transportation to another dimension of consciousness (Reichel-Dolmatoff, 1975, p. 35). The importance of the drugs has only been appreciated in recent decades, since anthropologists have begun to take them and report on their experiences (Harner, 1973, pp. 16ff; Reichel-Dolmatoff, 1971, p. 249, and 1975, pp. 118ff). Even modern Westerners have the experience of flying through space, traveling the Milky Way, meeting bird-headed people and talking dragons, and the like. No wonder, then, that preliterate peoples understand these experiences as attaining direct contact with a supernatural sphere and that the shaman, as the expert in attaining a controlled trance, is the translator and interpreter of this greater reality that surrounds and determines the events of everyday life.

If the foregoing be classified as the "cosmic" dimension of the shaman's trance, Iramamowe's task might be described in terms of a "transpersonal" dimension. He claims he can "see" that Texoma's soul is missing. In view of the universality of such a claim and to be consistent with our view that such formulations are serious attempts to describe real and familiar experiences, I believe we must grant that Iramamowe's report is factual. It may be metaphorical—as are the categories of every school of modern psychology; but it is an accurate attempt to describe a discrete experience. It is "transpersonal" in the sense that Iramamowe's impressions refer to the psychological condition of another individual, Texoma. *Transpersonal,* in this sense, refers to an experience whose meaning is not bounded by my personal existence. It transcends my personality and that of my partner. C. G. Jung (1946/1966) has discussed this phenomenon as the collective or archetypal dimension of the transference in his *Psychology of the Transference.* The western physician measures temperature, counts pulse, evaluates flushing and pallor, checks pupillary reflex—all sensory data in accordance with our very useful bias toward empirical evidence. These data are measurable with instruments. The shaman, however, evaluates the patient by means of feelings, intuitions, or imagination, data which are not so accessible to instrumentation. Yet we cannot dismiss the shaman's experience as "merely subjective," because—excepting the last century or so in the West—for millennia and apparently wherever human cultures have arisen, these transpersonal data have proven to be the only reliable source of diagnosis and cure.

Non-ordinary states of consciousness have also been the foundation upon which modern psychology has been built. Hypnosis, "hypnoid states," dreams, free association, active imagination, directed fantasy, and the like have been both tools for psychological investigation and models for theory-building. Transpersonal trance-like states, too, have been universally recognized as characteristic of the therapeutic relationship. Among the most unobtrusive of these would be the lowering of consciousness the therapist frequently experiences in the presence of the patient. For example, analysts who work with dreams report the phenomenon of being dumbfounded by the patient's dream imagery in the course of the session and yet find themselves quite capable of understanding the dream once the patient has left their office (Dieckmann, 1983, p. 51). Jung describes this as "contamination" or *"participation mystique,"* a term borrowed from anthropologist Lucien Lévy-Bruhl (1923/1966) and referring to a consciousness shared communally among the members of a preliterate society. Evidence of a "mystical participation" with the patient may very well appear in dreams. For example, I once dreamed of being aggressively seduced by a woman patient with whom I felt no particular erotic involvement at the conscious level. The perplexing element of the dream was that she had a penis. A couple of weeks later, however, she dreamed of being seduced by "the analyst," who was a lesbian.

We may conclude, then, that Iramamowe's transpersonal state is a kind of intense participation mystique which enables him to assess Texoma's condition. He experiences in feeling, image, or intuition, enough of her despondency to know that it is endangering her life. He directs his attention to his own unconscious in order to understand hers. With part of his psyche, he enters a mystical identity with her; and at the same time, with another part of his psyche, he retains his professional observer standpoint. We do this, in our own way, when we observe ourselves becoming stupid in the face of the patient's dream or caught by the patient's complex. We are stupid or caught because we are in a mystical participation with the patient, whose complex prevents him or her from understanding the dream or getting out of that stuckness. But we *know* we are being stupid or caught, and so we use our unconsciousness to take a sounding of the patient's complex.

When Iramamowe enters his trance and sees that Texoma's soul is missing, he experiences a void. He does not feel, image, or intuit her soul. There is nothing "in" her with which his drug-enhanced soul can connect. Though we moderns may be put off by the hide-and-seek imagery of disembodied souls, the imagery is consistent with our feelings in therapy with a patient. We cannot work with a patient if we cannot connect with something in him or her. That "something" in them and in us is what preliterate societies call "soul." For Texoma to be "without soul," means that the members of her community cannot connect with her. Iramamowe's diagnosis means that the community expert in maintaining sensitivity to this kind of connection has also failed; and the question is whether anyone can find and reestablish this connection before she dies.

Search for the Soul

In an account collected by Eliade (1971, pp. 19f), a Brazilian shaman hears a child's cry, investigates, and finds the soul of a sick girl in a recently harvested watermelon patch. We, too, sometimes feel ourselves presented with a visual or auditory fantasy which gives us the key to understanding a patient. It may be a rare experience for us, but it is typical in the sense that it occupies the sharp-focus end of a spectrum whose dimmer end fades into the unconscious. It typifies a feeling of intuitive certainty without which we have no conscious connection with the patient.

When Iramamowe announces that Texoma's soul is lost, he means he lacks this certainty. When he enlists the children and Donner to sweep the living area, he is asking whether any of them can find such certainty within themselves. The certainty is based on the same mystical participation which grounds all transpersonal connections between individuals. It appears in lovers when they find they are reading one another's minds. It manifests itself between us and our patients, for example, when patient A dreams a scene which apparently belongs to patient B's analysis—A and B being strangers, unaware of one another's existence. Such a coincidence can hardly be without meaning to the therapist. Very likely B's analysis has affected the therapist, and A's dream implies a conscious or unconscious sensitivity to this change. The important point, however, is that there are an infinite number of things about the therapist and about 20 or 30 other patients which A might have picked up on. This particular scene finds its way into the dream because it is highly important for A's psychology. The shaman would say that the dream shows us where A's soul has wandered—into B's melon patch.

One never knows what form such a "pointer" will take or when it will be encountered. This is why Iramamowe can say no more to Donner than that she will "just know" when she finds Texoma's soul. He has no idea whether it will be a feeling, an image, or an intuition that will occur with that distinctive certainty characteristic of establishing an inter-soul connection. As Donner tells the story, it is evident that she does not appreciate Iramamowe's words. She still does not know what it is she is looking for. Indeed, she does not even believe the soul is lost until she is overcome by that feeling of "indescribable helplessness" when Iramamowe turns to the sucking ritual.

Finding the Soul

Generally there are two theories of disease among American shamans: soul-loss and the intrusion of a pathogenic object, usually introduced by a hostile shaman (Eliade, 1951/1964, p. 300). Symptoms of intrusion disease are external injuries or internal pains, but with *no* ob-

101

vious changes in consciousness (Hultkrantz, 1967, p. 88). But Texoma is comatose; her consciousness has been drastically changed. Everyone knows her soul is lost, so why is Iramamowe acting as though this were a lesser disease? Anthropologist Donner has to have been aware of all this. The reason for her helplessness must be that Iramamowe seems to have given up the search for the soul.

Her helplessness reflects both her involvement in the Yanomama community and her awareness that the shaman's powers are failing him. She is more than an anthropologist, being a kind of "auntie" to the sick girl as well as a full-time participant in community life. She cannot be uninvolved. But in calling her helplessness "indescribable," Donner hints at its belonging to a different order of experience from that of personal involvement and observation. Something deeply unsettling jars her assessment of the situation. She realizes suddenly the earnestness of the Indians' concern. At this point she has not yet "found" the girl's soul in the full sense of making contact, and of being aware of that contact. But in the uncanny moment of helplessness, Donner is jolted into feeling the dire condition of things on a deeper plane.

Knowing at last that there is no time to lose, she immediately begins to act on a belief she has had all along, something related to her platitudes about the triviality of the girl's sickness. She becomes aware that the two nearly conflicting views of Texoma's illness are simultaneously true. The girl does have the flu, and must be treated for flu; yet that treatment must be pursued with the earnestness of a soul-restoring ritual. We encounter this as therapists when, for example, the patient's account of his or her anxiety is literally true and yet there is a "depth" to the account of which the patient is apparently ignorant and of whose nature we have only the vaguest glimmer. What we know for certain, in such a case, is only that "there is something there." That "something" is the soul the patient has lost; and our vague intimations are an indication of our transpersonal connection.

Iramamowe's questioning of Donner appears to be an attempt to assess her intuitive certainty. Is this hot-water cure the white woman's stupid attempt to deny the transpersonal; or is she, rather, grounded in the transpersonal? His anxiety on this score is also reflected later in his acute awareness of her faltering assurance before she utters the prayer. He needs to be sure that the healing work be grounded in a solid soul-to-soul connection. The ritual dimension of the cure is only important insofar as it articulates a feeling, image, or intuition of the patient's soul.

It is fortunate for us readers that Iramamowe found it in Donner, for this gives us a chance to witness the questioning process. We can identify with it as a necessary part of our work with patients. We must evaluate the validity, depth, and variety of our feelings for and intuitions about the patient. This is particularly true when we, like Iramamowe, are led by our countertransferential feelings outside the normal guidelines for therapy. For example, if we should get the notion with one particularly distressed narcissistic patient that it might be wise to accept phone calls, we need to be certain that our motivation does not proceed from mere sentimentality, from some savior complex in ourselves, or the like. It must be justified by a differentiated grasp of the state of the patient's soul, or by our certain awareness of where the soul has wandered.

There are at least three components to the countertransferential connection Donner has with Texoma. First there is the intuition that her sickness is "only the flu": This intimation of easy curability seems in retrospect to be evidence that Texoma's soul was never wholly lost, in that one member of the community (Donner) had never lost her connection with it. This despite the fact that Donner remained for a long time unconscious of the connection. Secondly, Donner's feeling of helplessness makes her conscious of the seriousness of the situation. It may be that she has finally tuned in to the collective mentality of the community. But it may as well be that that "indescribable helplessness" is what Fordham (1978) calls a "syntonic" countertransferential feeling: that she feels the same despair Texoma felt when she was last conscious. It may be that the state of Texoma's soul is found precisely in this feeling. Thirdly, Donner has the memory of her grandmother's cure for the flu. This memory identifies her with the sick girl—she knows what it feels like to be sick this way and to be treated properly. These three components of Donner's countertransference are essential elements in any successful cure: a recognition of where the patient's soul has wandered (in this case, despair and helplessness); a realization of how near it is to home (Donner's intuition that it is "only flu"); and an orientedness whereby one can find the path or blaze the trail over which the soul can be led. Regarding this last point, shamans in preliterate cultures speak of learning the topography of the transcendent world; for Donner it is the grandmother's cure.

Restoring the Soul

In the story of the Brazilian shaman who finds the soul of a sick girl in a melon patch, he restores it when he places it "on the child's head and strokes it down her body." For us this may be a quaint story, because we have no notion of how an immaterial substance can be "stroked" into a material substance. We cannot imagine how this relates to the psychotherapy we do. Donner's experience is much easier to understand because although the image of stroking cannot be "felt" the way a psychotherapist feels, the grandmother cure can be.

Donner's cure is rich with implications we can readily appreciate. In the first place it is an effective social ritual, for it engages all the people

103

most closely connected with the sick girl and gives them something to do to express their love and concern. All the frustrated longings to assist on the parts of Texoma's "mothers" (her own mother and her father's second wife) and grandmothers are harnessed in the preparation of hot compresses while her playmates are engaged in fire-tending and palm-frond heating. We moderns can hardly understand Texoma's loss of soul apart from the familial and social implications of the dangerous raid in which Texoma's father may have lost his life and in reaction to which her mother seems to have drifted into depression—perhaps has been in danger of losing her own soul. Furthermore, the whole community, bereft of its best warriors, must feel itself in a kind of twilight state between life and death. Donner's cure therefore not only works to "convince" the sick girl that she is loved and valuable, it also energizes the community and gives it a reason to exist.

On the other hand, the cure makes excellent sense when we look at it in terms of Donner's countertransference. It appears that she allows herself to identify with Texoma, to feel the depression and helplessness and the longing to be cared for. This activates memories from her own childhood when she was sick like Texoma. The cure is designed on the basis of these memories because it is the obvious "pathway" from the "found" state of Texoma's soul (abandonment and annihilation) to its potential restoration ("only flu"). By treating Texoma simultaneously as though she has the flu and yet with the solemnity and transcendental awareness appropriate to her lost-soul condition, Donner "strokes" the soul back into the girl. In order to accomplish this kind of a restoration of soul, the psychotherapist must find the patient's pathology within him- or herself—much as a stage actor cannot function unless he or she can find the character within and develop it into a full-blown personality. Jungians sometimes speak in this context of "the wounded healer" (Sammuels, 1985, pp. 187-191).

Another way we could formulate Donner's cure is to say that she restores Texoma's "will to live," which is one of the common ways Westerners have used to characterize what preliterate people mean by *soul*. It implies that the will to live may be lost but recoverable if it has not "strayed too far." This is the condition of our patients who have become lost in a plethora of events, obligations, and expectations, pulling them this way and that. Sometimes—all too rarely—we are fortunate enough to see right through the confusion and grasp the very nature of the patient's will to live. This can occasion a magical course of therapy in which we seem to do little more than watch and listen as the patient pulls everything together almost singlehandedly. Such patients tell us that no one has ever "heard" them before, they owe their progress all to us. It is true; we *have* heard them in a uniquely efficacious way. To understand everything they say in terms of a less-than-conscious core of the personality is to understand it better than they do themselves.

When Donner's assurance falters and she utters a prayer, it is as though she has switched levels and can no longer understand how a grandmother cure could work. Iramamowe's anxiety evidently asks the implicit question, "Has the soul slipped away from you, or are you only indulging in your white woman's penchant for denying the transpersonal? Her oscillating certainty corresponds to Jung's (1937/1966) in the case of a woman who had dreams involving extravagant symbolism that mystified him. His suggestion that they quit the charade of therapy was met with firm refusal, as very important effects were being felt. Some time after the symbolic process had completed itself, Jung found a close parallel to the woman's dreams in the symbolism of kundalini yoga. Inasmuch as in Jung's writings the finding of the patient's soul is usually demonstrated through confident interpretation of the patient's symbolism, it appears that Jung had found the soul of his patient but—like Donner—could not make the finding conscious. Like Iramamowe with Texoma, Jung had not the patience or courage to go on with the kundalini woman without being sure he has found her soul. It is an indication of how far out on a limb Donner has gone. *We* know that both Donner and Jung had found their patients' souls, but *they* did not.

Donner brings herself back to a dim awareness of the transpersonal connection by mumbling a prayer with childlike fervor. She is confused by the mixture of "magic, religion, and fear" because, through the development of her anthropologist's ego with its critical, rational power, she has come to devalue her childish associations. They are indeed inadequate for scientific research, but this does not mean they are in all ways inferior. If they lead us to a relatively undifferentiated, childish way of thinking, they are also leading us to a mystical participation with the world and with other individuals: the very ground of the soul-soul connection. In Donner's case, it is likely that the hot-compress cure, the security of grandmother's competence, the power of God to make things right, and the earliest infant-parent bond, all belong to the same complex of memories; and that this is the essence of what Texoma has lost in losing her soul. Thus Donner's prayer appears to be an appeal to the divine and familial source of infantile security. It is tempting (even if unscientific) to wonder whether this prayer—almost alone—may not have restored Texoma's soul. It blazes a trail from soul-banishing despair to the soul-restoring security of the ultimate.

Conclusion

Levi-Strauss (1956/1967) retells Franz Boas' story of the Kwakiutl shaman, Quesalid, who, as a youth, believes shamanism to be fakery and therefore studies with shamans in order to expose them. Ironically, he becomes known as a truly great shaman; for he exposes others by curing the patients with whom they have failed, using techniques learned from foreign shamans, which patient, failed shaman, and community have never before seen. At times it seems that Quesalid believes his own cures to consist in trickery. In this context, Donner's cure may be seen as a kind of noncynical and unconscious trickery that achieves its effects by a symbolism more dramatically apt than anything the Yanomama have ever seen. This explanation, however leaves much to be desired. For one thing, how do we explain Texoma's recovery, as she has been unconscious throughout the cure and beyond the reach of the drama? If we speculate that the change effected by the symbolism in community consciousness must have been transmitted to the girl despite her comatose condition, we open the door again to a soul-soul hypothesis. Quesalid, too, by the end of his life, seems to have been ready to grant that shamans who do not fall victim to the lure of self-aggrandizement may be "genuine."

I have been led to the model of soul-loss and soul-restoration by a series of cures or partial cures for which I have been able to find no ordinary explanation. I have mentioned fragments from some of these in the course of this paper. Most extraordinary is the case of a woman who came regularly to weekly sessions over a period of more than 2 years and sat in total silence for the vast majority of them. Mindful of Jung's experience with the kundalini woman, I was careful only to ascertain from time to time whether she was satisfied with the way things were going. Near the end of her course of sittings, she detailed for me some of the very impressive changes that had taken place in her life. Like Donner, I had had only the vaguest of hints that we were on the right track—or, indeed, on any track at all.

REFERENCES

Dieckmann, H. (1983). Die Deutung des Traums in der Analyse. *Zeitschrift für analytische Psychologie und ihre Grenzgebiete, 14*(1), 50-64.

Donner, F. (1982). *Shabono.* New York: Delacorte.

Eliade, M. (1964). In W. Trask (Trans.), *Shamanism: Archaic techniques of ecstasy.* New York: Pantheon. (Original work published 1951).

Eliade, M. (1969). In W. Trask (Trans.), *Yoga, immortality and freedom.* Princeton: Princeton University Press. (Original work published 1954).

Eliade, M. (1971). *From medicine men to Muhammad: A thematic source book of the history of religions.* New York: Harper & Row.

Fordham, M. (1978). *Jungian psychotherapy.* New York: Wiley.

Harner, M. (1973). The sound of rushing water. In M. Harner (Ed.), *Hallucinogens and shamanism* (pp. 15-27). New York: Oxford University Press.

Hultkrantz, A. (1967). In M. Setterwall (Trans.), *The religions of the American Indians.* Berkeley: University of California Press.

Jung, C. (1960). Basic postulates of analytical psychology. In H. Read, M. Fordham, & G. Adler (Eds.) and R. Hull (Trans.), *The collected works of C. G.*

Jung (Vol. 8, pp. 338-357). New York: Pantheon. (Original work published 1931).

Jung, C. (1964). Mind and earth. In H. Read, M. Fordham, & G. Adler (Eds.) and R. Hull (Trans.), *The collected works of C. G. Jung* (Vol. 10, pp. 29-49). New York: Pantheon. (Original work published 1927).

Jung, C. (1966a). The realities of practical psychotherapy. In H. Read, M. Fordham, & G. Adler (Eds.) and R. Hull (Trans.), *The collected works of C. G. Jung* (Vol. 16, pp. 327-338). New York: Pantheon. (Original lecture delivered 1937).

Jung, C. (1966b). The psychology of the transference. In H. Read, M. Fordham, & G. Adler (Eds.) and R. Hull (Trans.), *The collected works of C. G. Jung* (Vol. 16, pp. 163-323). New York: Pantheon. (Original work published 1946).

Jung, C. (1969). Concerning rebirth. In H. Read, M. Fordham, G. Adler, & W. McGuire (Eds.), and R. Hull (Trans.), *The collected works of C. G. Jung* (Vol. 9₁). Princeton: Princeton University Press. (Original work published 1939).

Jung, C. (1971). *Psychological types,* In H. Read, M. Fordham, G. Adler, & W. McGuire (Eds.) and H. Baynes, revised by R. Hull (Trans.), *The collected works of C. G. Jung* (Vol. 6). Princeton: Princeton University Press. (Original work published 1921).

Lévi-Strauss, C. (1967). The sorcerer and his magic. In C. Jacobson & B. Schoepf (Trans.), *Structural anthropology* (pp. 161-180). Garden City, NY: Doubleday. (Original work published 1958).

Lévy-Bruhl, L. (1966). *Primitive mentality* (L. Claire, Trans.). Boston: Beacon. (Original work published 1923).

Nowak, M. (1977). Introduction. In M. Nowak & S. Durrant, *The tale of the Nisan shamaness* (pp. 3-38). Seattle: University of Washington Press.

Reichel-Dolmatoff, G. (1971). *Amazonian cosmos: The sexual and religious symbolism of the Tukano Indians.* Chicago: University of Chicago Press.

Reichel-Dolmatoff, G. (1975). *The shaman and the jaguar: A study of narcotic drugs among the Indians of Colombia.* Philadelphia: Temple University Press.

Sammuels, A. (1985). *Jung and the post-Jungians.* Boston: Routledge & Kegan Paul.

Underhill, R. (1968). *Red man's religion: Beliefs and practices of the Indians north of Mexico.* Chicago: University of Chicago Press.

Van der Leeuw, G. (1963). *Religion in essence and manifestation* (Vol. 1), J. Turner (Trans.). New York: Harper & Row. (Original work published 1933).

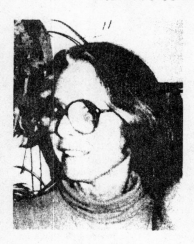

Nan Wolcott

We the Alchemists of the Soul

A Leo of August sun and moons, I was born in Stockbridge, Massachusetts and grew up on Staten Island in view of the dazzle of New York City where I now live and practice when I am not: with my blossoming family in Vermont (6 children; 14 grandchildren) or attending transformational seminars and world travels with Drs. Jean Houston and Robert Masters. Studies: Columbia-Presbyterian Hospital, R.N.; Union Graduate School, Ph.D.; initial Jungian studies at the University of Vermont's Religion Department.

142 West 82 Street #5
New York, New York 10024

Jung spent the last 30 years of his life exploring and documenting the symbolism of alchemy, the main contribution of his lifetime. Alchemy was not a search for gold per se, but a search for the golden opportunity, the gold in the person, the unknown in the psyche as well as the unknown in matter. This was new knowledge for the alchemists, as it is for us through Jung, and contained a religious numinosity that created psychic rumblings. Alchemy presents psychic contents in a historical context. The alchemist's *opus* was the projection of properties onto matter as the alchemist experienced the eruption of the contents of his own unconscious. What occurred was the symbolic externalization of the objective psyche, the collective unconscious and the changes this psyche undergoes. The alchemist's recorded images concretized the images from the collective unconscious, uncovering, discovering, and dissecting its anatomy.

"Have you ever read *Man and his Symbols?*" "No," I answered, "Who wrote it?" I was a student at Goddard College doing my first semester in sculpture. A faculty member, a psychologist, posed the question that was to change the course of my studies, the contents of my dreams, and the path of my life. I switched my major to psychology pursuing C. G. "Yung" but my proposal was almost refused because I couldn't spell his name. Now, a timeless time later, my Ph.D. in Social and Clinical Psychology based on many disciplines is behind me, along with 7 years—a magic number—of Jungian analysis. I have seen a multitude of clients on the job and in private practice. I can now reflect upon the meaning Jung's work has had upon my journey of individuation, my being in the world, my relationships, my practice, my psyche dreaming on toward healing and wholeness. A potent core of Jung's work for me has been his volumes on alchemy, a subject still rather infrequently recognized, written about, or discussed. What follows are alchemical condensations that I (Wolcott, 1979) have written pertaining to the alchemy of psychotherapy based on six lectures given by Edward Edinger, M.D. (1968).

Alchemy is an operational mythology and its symbolism represents procedures to bring about changes as psychotherapy is operational in the same way. In alchemy and psychotherapy the undifferentiated stuff from which comes the birth of consciousness is the *prima materia*. It represents first matter and the image of the child, the self, in a place of pure potency and with an indeterminate power of change. In order to transform matter it must be reduced to the undifferentiated, innocent, original state, freeing up rigid patterns of being in order to change, to become transformed. "Become like children," said Jesus. *Prima materia* is not made, you have to find it in the nooks and crannies of ordinary life. It has many names but is one thing: the psychology of our own multiplicity with one underlying unity. The *opus,* the holy work, requires waiting, enduring, tolerance, courage, and patience. Insights gained in psychotherapy are not derived from *deserving* them or *earning* them but are received with a sense of grace, as a gift of God. It is an inner task that may alienate one from the world which does not have a healthy relationship to the individual's subjective side. Yet the work as the alchemist's *opus,* is a secret not to be shared with the inadept and contains a profound sense of mystery emphasizing the worth of the individual versus the collective. Transformation should not be given hard and fast names, leaving interpretation open to flexibility, as twilight is dispelled by too much clarity. Our own secrets or those of our clients must remain open to this flexibility in the process of psychotherapy.

The Operations of Psychotherapy and Alchemy

1. *Calcinatio* is the chemical process of calcination, an intense drying out of all constituents that are volatile. The alchemists gave fire symbols to calcium unaware of the similarity of happenings when a fire of libido intensity is applied to a psychic substance. They equated fire with love, with God, as He burned with divine love. By fire, imperfection is driven away, burned up, melted, separated, leaving the solid. The fire of bereavement, the frustration of the desires of lust, greed, and possessive love are related to developing the individuated Self through the frustration of these very same desires.

In psychological transformations one must seek objects away from the anima and the animus, away from *concupiscentia,* desirousness, in which you allow yourself to be led down the path of self-indulgence by them. This allowance is the fire of heaven or hell in which we become possessed by the anima/animus object. If we can say "I don't have to get it," put it aside as the alchemists put their substances in the crucible, with the firm thought that it was the right thing to do, then we become quiet and change. It may be uncomfortable, the devil may rumble, but self-control and non-indulgence will become a habit. There will be growth. The stone, the alchemist's gold, the philosopher's stone, is growing and the stone will be a diamond.

After a *calcinatio* experience you become immune to it. Witness a shaman swallowing a fire. Psychologically we become immune to intense emotional affect. If we act upon the *nigredo,* the alchemist's dung, the black, dark, shadow side of our personalities, it turns white becoming purified. *Slake* lime undergoes purgatorial rejuvenation becoming quick lime, from which develops white, purified ash.

Therapeutically, *calcinatio* is a drying out of waterlogged psychic contents, a drying out of unconscious complexes. Fire resides in the complex, becoming conscious when made known to the therapist. The fire of consciousness dries up. The complex cleaning up the unconscious contamination.

2. *Solutio* is the chemical operation that turns everything to water. The goal is to dissolve and coagulate. A taken-for-granted experience for us, the alchemist considered it a remarkable, wondrous phenomenon that you could add a solid substance, salt for instance, to a solvent, usually water, and it disappears. He got so caught up in the wonder of this vanishing act that it attraced all kinds of images to him which he then projected on this operation.

Alchemists wrote of Sol and Luna dissolving in the material waters, the maternal womb. Sol, as gold, and Luna, as silver, dissolve in mercury, and as it amalgamates with them they disappear. Using crude pulverized ore, they would dissolve it in mercury, and boil off the mercury, leaving pure gold behind. This was a chemical procedure, yet the alchemists used terms such as mother, womb, born again, superimposing components of the psyche, psychological images. Sol, as the masculine ego and Luna, as the anima, became united in the friendly water, mercury, returning to the maternal womb, the *prima materia,* the maternal water from which they came. Symbolically, this is incest, a return to the unconscious, a re-dissolution, to be purified, regenerated, reborn in a new form from the source from which one came.

In summary, the psychological implications of *solutio* are:

a. The analytical process is a "lysis," a loosening and separating process. One must confront consciousness with the unconsciousness' statement, which can loosen up rigid attitudes through clarification of dreams in analysis. Rigid ego attitudes must die or be released in order to reach the proper *solutio* for the soul, the psyche.

b. The containing solvent is a more comprehensive attitude. As one explores the unconscious, the self, the totality of the personality is realized. The adult, like a child, is in sympathy with the solvent, like the mother, and yearns to be contained by it, affecting a real feeling quality of wanting to be held and nurtured. Through therapy, any psychological attitude embodies a union of a pair of opposites, one being more comprehensive and one being lesser. This union of a pair of opposites, as experienced by an analysand, could be therapy itself as the containing solvent, the more comprehensive attitude, while the lesser attitude is one of resistance and denial.

c. Consider the properties of liquids. They flow in a fixed volume but have no fixed shape. They are soft and fluid. If you pour them into a container they seek the lowest level; if they meet an obstacle they flow around it. This is expressive of the fluidity between client and therapist. Every unconscious content and complex contains its own water which will dissolve them. The "water" represents the dreams that emanate from the unconscious complex describing its contents; and the spirit of understanding, the potentiality of consciousness.

3. *Coagulatio* refers to solidification. A solid is dissolved when evaporated and reappears again, precipitating out. Water cooled becomes ice; molten metal cooling becomes solidified; an egg becomes coagulated when cooked. *Coagulatio* turns substance into earth which is stable, reliable, durable, non-volatile.

The alchemists wrote about coagulating quicksilver in sulphur which does not burn. Of course sulphur burns. They meant "philosophical" sulphur that is connected with the sun. It is fiery, inflammable, yellow, gold. It is also the devil, evil, smelly. It corrupts and it blackens all metals. Sulphur coagulates all, representing consciousness, will, and compulsion and the involuntary desirousness. The word proportional means the relationship of one entity to another; analogy is a separate but inner relatedness. Analogy coagulates. Depth psychology as an operational procedure is a treasury of analogies that coagulate and corporify the objective psyche and the processes it undergoes in development. The analogy gives form and visibility to the intangible, to the uncoagulated, and to that which was unrealized. Concepts and abstraction do not coagulate. They make air, not earth. Images and myths, the stuff of the soul, coagulate the outer world with the inner world. Affective images toss us about until they coagulate and we can view them objectively. "The word made flesh" is in itself a symbolic expression of the process. It is an analogy which helps coagulate, give form to the nature of the psychic process and the task of becoming real. Creation, solid matter, emerged out of chaos. The creation of a psychic content does not occur until that content is coagulated.

For the alchemists, mercury was the "fugitive slave" with an evasive quality that had to be fixed, held down by amalgamating it with magnesium or sulphur in order that it become solid. Within the personality there are certain aspects of the psyche that are not materialized or apprehendable in any particular form. The energy of psychic complexes hits you or an emerging insight flashes into consciousness and then it is gone. They need to be fixed or coagulated. They become fixed only by relating them to black, ordinary reality. The black component, our shadow side of our personality, must be integrated. We have to be solid in order to cast a shadow.

Coagulatio is the process of particularization, realization, and concretization. An analogy coagulates and makes the connection with one's inner relatedness, belonging to the status of introversion. Proportion is the relationship toward the outward belonging to the state of extroversion.

4. *Sublimatio* and *separatio*. *Sublimatio* occurs when mercury, sulphur, or any solid substance is heated in the bottom of a vessel to a gaseous state, sublimates off, re-collecting at the top of the vessel. This conception of sublimation is obviously a totally opposite one to that of Freud. The word comes from the Latin word *sublime,* meaning high; the process of elevating. *Sublimatio,* similar to the process of distillation, is the operation in which a lower substance, of a lower realm, is elevated or raised. A solid becomes vaporized, volatized, impalpable, invisible. In corresponding psychological effects, the lower that is of little esteem becomes uppermost in importance. The alchemist illustrated this particular *opus* by a white dove flying upward within the vessel. The vessel has a cosmic significance. The lower part represents earth and the upper dome the heavens. The fugitive from the lower part took off and flew to the heavenly realm, transporting itself to heaven. The alchemist liberates the *anima mundi* imprisoned in matter. He experienced constant suffering and the need for redemption. He sought the liberation of the world soul in the darkness of matter, in the unconscious, where it lives in latency. He did not seek his own salvation through the grace of God but through the liberation of God from the darkness of matter.

Psychologically, of central value here is the Self as God, redeemed from the darkness of the unconscious in its state of latency. The ego's relationship to the transpersonal is important. The ascent, the rising above, the elevating process gives one distance and perspective from all the entanglements of the particular and all its earthly, personalistic details. The higher one goes the better the view, but it also can be remote. *Sublimatio,* the generalization and the abstraction of all kinds, releases many caged birds. It has a deep archetypal, universal meaning and cannot be imposed arbitrarily without its mythological content. In the process of therapy the same matter, the same problems arise, recirculating through our alchemist's vessel. Only gradually does the purifying and solidifying come into realization. Ascent and descent dreams are common for analysands. When one is "above" the problem some objectivity can be achieved.

Separatio has a more general rather than specific reference to any chemical procedure. It is the process of extracting a metal from its crude ore, dividing it from its earthly dross. The undifferentiated mixture undergoes differentiation. The symbolic implications are those of order and distinctness versus disorder and a confused state. The individual's soul becomes extracted in the particular form that confronts us. That particular form has lost its libido content because we have extracted its meaning. It is no longer alive with our projected meaning. Emerging psychological contents come up with trailing contaminations, impure and undifferentiated. We must clean them up and separate them from things to which they do not belong. They must be attenuated, reduced to a fine powder as they recirculate again and again. This is not a final end but a beginning, or an intermediate state that is required before *coniunctio.*

5. *Mortificatio, putreficatio,* and *coniunctio.*

Mortificatio and *putrefacatio* are two factors of the same thing which represent the tendency of alchemists, to project completely, not unlike ourselves, and to personify the materials they were working with. *Mortificatio* literally means killing or making dead. It can be related to religious asceticism that concerns itself with the subjection of appetites, penance, abstinence, and painful afflictions on the body. The human being is in the flask and the torturing of the material is the torturing of the human body.

Putrefactio is the rotting and decomposition of bodies and is the most negative of all alchemical procedures. It symbolizes blackness, *nigredo,* dismemberment, death, humiliation, mutilation. The images are powerful and grisly but there are positive, transformational images clustered about, such as resurrection, regeneration, and rebirth.

In both *mortificatio* and *putrefactio* blackness is a very prominent symbol. "Black" is the beginning of "white" and a sign of putrefication and alteration in the body. Psychologically this is the *sine qua non* of the therapeutic process. "Integrate the shadow" is a quiet statement but one has images that are not so quiet but rather very alarming. Putrefication and mortification precede every new form that comes into consciousness.

The negative becomes positive; there is a union of opposites. *Felix culpa:* Adam's sin was a happy one because redemption can take place constituting a transformation. The ego must be promoted but it also must be purified.

There is a lesser *coniunctio,* an intermediate process indicating that more development is needed; and a greater *coniunctio,* which is the final goal of the *opus.*

The greater *coniunctio* is the phenomenology of the self. It is the union of opposites, the marriage of contraries. The constellation of opposites means for those who experience it distress and paralysis and then a release through both of the opposites. These are very abstract, and innocuous ideas when expressed verbally, but each person must experience what this means out of the vital stuff of his or her own life and its agonizing reality. But in the midst of this conflict an understanding of the philosopher's stone, *lapis philosophorum* is helpful. There are many different terms for the *lapis philosophorum.* The term itself implies the opposite. Philosophy is the love of wisdom and from the beginning of its existence it represented a spiritual endeavor. A stone is the hardest of realities. It is concrete. It is the concrete, practical, realistic efficacy of psychic stuff called consciousness. The alchemical definition, "a stone that is not a stone," is a contradiction in itself. The stone is a substance which is petrine as regards its efficacy and virtue, but not as regards its substance. The nature of the stone is unconscious nature, as Christ's spirituality; and the reality of the psyche, which is hard, durable, and eternal. The spirit is fixed in the eternal stone. Intuitively and intellectually, the alchemists brought the Greek philosophers' insights into concrete realization. For Christianity, the alchemists gave symbols, concretization, to the insights of Plato and the Stoics, making available to a multitude that which otherwise would have been inaccessible to them.

Multiplicatio is a characteristic of the stone. It might be the image that is projected upon the inferior material and the stone multiplies. This is an interesting quality, psychologically speaking. Similarly *proiectio* presumes that consciousness is contagious and has a self-multiplying tendency. The wholeness of the personality has a self-multiplying tendency. In the process of psychotherapy consciousness can be contagious if there is openness between the therapist and client. The personality of the therapist in relationship to the patient is more important than anything the therapist says. The therapist must be susceptible to the personality of the patient. It is a reciprocal process. You can exert no influence if you are not susceptible to influence. The reciprocal qualities of the stone stem from the fact that the qualities of the whole and centered personality only exist in relationship to the source of life. As the ego pays serious attention to the unconscious, it, in turn reciprocates and a mutual *opus* is formed just as the latent philosopher's stone present in the *prima materia* needs the devoted conscious efforts of the ego in order to come into actuality. Together they work, as therapist and client work, on the grand undertaking, leading through the aforementioned stages of alchemy towards the individuating self and a *coniunctio,* to create more and more consciousness in the universe. The goal of the *opus* is the goal of a lifetime. But the essential thing is the journey of life, the *opus* which leads to the goal.

> If thou knowest how to moisten this dry earth with its own water, thou wilt loosen the pores of earth.

> If you will contemplate your lack of fantasy, of inspiration and inner aliveness, which you feel as sheer stagnation and a barren wilderness, and impregnate it with the interest born of alarm at your inner death, then something can take shape in you, for your inner emptiness conceals just as great a fullness if only you will allow it to penetrate into you. If you prove receptive to this "call of the wild," the longing for fulfillment will quicken the sterile wilderness of your soul as rain quickens the dry earth.

Alchemical Text of Philaletha's (Jung, 1955/1963)

REFERENCES

Edinger, E. (1968). *Psychotherapy and the stages of alchemy.* Taped lectures available at the Kristine Mann Library, the C. G. Jung Foundation, New York, NY. Later published in six issues of the *Quadrant,* quarterly magazine of the C. G. Jung Foundation, New York, NY.

Jung, C. G. (1963). Mysterium coniunctionis. In H. Read, M. Fordham, & G. Adler (Eds.) and R. Hull (Trans.), *The collected works of C. G. Jung* (Vol. 14). New York: Pantheon/Bollingen Series XX. (Original work published 1955).

Wolcott, N. D. (1979). *Alchemy and alcoholism based on the psychology of C. G. Jung.* Ann Arbor, MI: University Microfilms International.

Henry Elkin
E. Mark Stern

Toward a Freud-Jung Reconciliation

An Interview

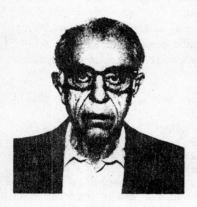

301 East 87 Street
New York, New York 10128

Henry Elkin received his Ph.D. in Anthropology from Columbia University in 1941. He studied at the C. G. Jung Institute in Zurich from 1951 to 1955. He was a Council Member of the Association of Existential Psychology and Psychiatry, and Co-Editor of the *Review of Existential Psychology and Psychiatry*. Dr. Elkin has been Professor of Psychology at Duquesne University in Pittsburgh, faculty member of the Washington School of Psychiatry, and Lecturer at the New School for Social Research in New York City. He regards the development of his whole pattern of thought as reflecting his experience of World War II. He is in private practice in New York City.

E. Mark Stern: I know you studied in Zurich, knew Carl Gustav Jung, maybe even had sessions with him. Yet you don't quite come across as a Jungian, or like other Jungians I know. Do you consider yourself a Jungian?

Henry Elkin: I was made honorary member of the London, England, "Society of Analytic Psychology" back in 1971 when an article of mine appeared that they used in their training program. That's my only formal Jungian affiliation, of which I'm very proud. Like myself, they've been strongly influenced by the British, original "object relations" approach, especially by the work of Melanie Klein. Also like myself, they were generally viewed as heretical by other Jungians. It's only recently that I've discovered that their kind of nonsectarian approach has been taken over in part by a growing number of Jungians, especially in the San Francisco area and even by at least one outstanding Jungian in Zurich, Mario Jacobi. So I'm delighted to feel more at home myself in the Jungian world.

EMS: Why did you get involved with the Jungian approach to begin with?

HE: I got my Ph.D. in anthropology when "culture and personality" was the big thing. Margaret Mead, Ruth Benedict, Gregory Bateson, and others turned to Freudian theory for enlightenment on this subject. I saw, and still see, Jungian theory as the better *anthropology,* in its original pre-Darwinian sense of "science of man."

EMS: How so? Can you put that in perspective?

HE: Because Jung recognized the foundational role of the mother in human psychic life and appreciated what I call the mystical-religious dimension of the psyche, which I saw as grounded on the infant's experience. For I was already familiar with the research of René Spitz, Arnold Gesell, and others in 1951 when I arrived in Zurich. The foundational role of the mother-child relation is now widely accepted, but only Jung gives due acknowledgment to its mystical-religious aspect.

EMS: Are you referring to Jung's (1952) *Answer to Job,* where he speaks of the Roman Catholic Pope's proclaiming the dogma of the Blessed Mother's bodily assumption into heaven? Jung spoke of this as the most important affirmation of our time because it noted that the feminine principle had finally been recognized as joining the male Godhead.

HE: Yes, but it's just with the appearance of that book that I began to have misgivings about Jung. For it made me see why his appreciation of the mystical-religious realm tended to get bogged down by intellectual mystification and foster what I'd call the peculiarly Jungian form of therapeutic psychopathy.

EMS: How do you mean that?

HE: He attributed mystical-religious experience to the *collective unconscious,* which was OK by me. But he regarded this as biologically, racially inherited and as completely separate and distinct from the *personal unconscious,* the individual's actual developmental experience. It's this sharp bifurcation that's given rise to an underlying and all-pervasive intellectual mystification that has closed Jungians off, until recently, from dialogue with those belonging to other schools of therapy. It all followed from Jung's staking out his own claim as the master of the collective unconscious over against Freud, whom he regarded as the master of the personal unconscious.

EMS: But where does the psychopathy come in?

HE: That came up because you mentioned *Answer to Job.* There he speaks of the archetypal shadow as the evil, satanic part of God.

EMS: To what extent did the notion of shadow both aid the whole Jungian system and how at the same time might it have created a level of doubt or dishonesty?

HE: The shadow is perhaps Jung's greatest, most useful single working concept. But reducing it ultimately to this "archetypal shadow" serves to justify the acceptance and practice of one's own evil, under the guise of achieving Divine "wholeness." This may well serve one's creative and destructive effectiveness in the world. But it is directly counter to the principles underlying all higher civilization, and betokens a fall-back into what I call modern primitivism, a form of mindlessness characteristic of our own time. Jung may well have been prophetic on this score, but he surely would have deplored this outcome.

EMS: It's interesting because another person picked this up. It was Victor White, an English Dominican priest. In his correspondence he really took Jung to task. His book *Soul and Psyche* (White, 1960) was a response to *Answer to Job*. In it he faulted Jung's misunderstanding of evil as a corporeal manifestation. White espoused the concept of evil as the absence of good, just as darkness is the absence of light.

HE: I certainly went along with Victor White on this score. In fact, if *Answer to Job* had already appeared, I perhaps would not have gone to Zurich.

EMS: Didn't Jung see Hitler ultimately as the personification of evil?

HE: He certainly was anti-Hitler—after the first couple of years in any case. But I don't know if he necessarily saw him as any special personification of evil.

EMS: In his letters he actually does refer to him in that way. Apparently he couldn't account for the Nazi regime in any other way. He needed to see evil personified. He becomes polarized. That's not process. Where you you take this, Henry?

HE: For me, the problem of evil, the moral and ethical problem, must be seen in terms of infantile development. The baby is confronted with a moral problem at 8 months of age. Melanie Klein (Segal, 1979) puts guilt at 3 months. I think she's wrong, but at 8 months of age, in agreement with D. W. Winnicott (1965) and in accord with René Spitz's (1965) and others' empirical research, that child certainly knows guilt. It's right there.

EMS: But it's the guilt of the savage, the criminal, the murderer.

HE: One of the terms I often use is "baby killer." Every baby is a killer, as in a temper tantrum. I myself think that no therapy has ever been resolved at its core unless it deals with the baby killer. Neither Primal Therapy nor Bioenergetics can deal with it effectively because they don't see the baby's rage as linked to the corresponding guilt. Melanie Klein was the first to see their inherent linkage.

EMS: If Melanie Klein had been a Jungian rather than a Freudian, what would you think of her importance?

HE: The fact that Melanie Klein started out, not with Freud in Vienna, but in Budapest with Sandor Ferenczi, helps account for her great innovations. Freud and Ferenczi finally broke with one another. Melanie Klein found a real home in England.

EMS: So we're really dealing with the birth of rapprochement—a new underground linking Jung and Klein.

HE: Not just Jung and Klein. I recently heard Joseph Sandler, the distinguished protégé of Anna Freud, propose that the term "id" be replaced in psychoanalytic thinking by the concept of "the inner child."

What I'm most grateful for in my Jungian training is the way I've learned to work with dreams. Freud called dream interpretation "the royal road to the unconscious." But his way of interpreting dreams took no account of the basic principles by which the unconscious mind works. Dreams reflect the operations of the preverbal human mind which deals mainly with visual images. Everything I say about the first year of life can be demonstrated by dream operations. Jung's great achievement was to devise a truly phenomenological—properly scientific—*formal* method of dream interpretation, such as was later hit upon by Fairbairn and by the outstanding Kleinian, Donald Meltzer (1983). But it's Jung's practice of dream interpretation that most tellingly reveals his own form of therapeutic psychopathy. He never systematically related the meanings he found in his patients' dreams to the transference situation. For that would have undermined the great Guru role he played with his followers.

EMS: Do you have a clinical example of how the dream becomes a stepping stone to that first year of life?

HE: The first thing that comes to mind is a patient that I saw only yesterday. He dreamed of getting to the top floor of a building where he'd never been before, looks out of a window, and sees an elevated railroad station that is no longer operative and is being taken down. The meaning was very clear. Riding in a train is a collective action in contrast to walking, or riding a bicycle, for example. An elevated railway means collective spirituality, taking over as if by contagion the ideas and values of his surroundings. He had no truly personal autonomous mental-spiritual life. Now he sees that this elevated station is being dismantled. I know that what's happening is that I'm helping to bring the guy down to earth, into his own bodily nature, back from being swept along by collective ideas and trendy fads.

EMS: How does that relate specifically to the first year of life?

HE: This particular patient was very much his mother's son. He still is hooked on his mother-goddess image. And his only recourse—freedom, autonomy for him—is art work. He has a real artistic gift. But his ideological outlook on life, so to speak, the way he sees human and social relations and everything else—he's not autonomous whatsoever. He just sort of picks up the ideas, that latest fad that prevails in his social surroundings. It's the elevated railway, you see. In some sense, what we have to do with this patient is to achieve a mental-spiritual orientation whereby his artistic gifts will truly express his personal being.

There are better examples. Here is another one of a couple of days ago. The patient dreams of entering my actual building. He gets into the elevator which here is like that on a construction job, with no walls, along with a gang of workmen. Also in this elevator is a very attractive young woman, a pregnant whore. I know from this dream that his therapy is about to enter into its final stage. First of all, the analytic situation is portrayed as a construction job. *Analysis, as I see it, is a deconstruction and reconstruction job.* The workmen symbolize the collective non-personal aspects of his masculine being. The pregnant whore symbolizes his original, mother-identified *female* side—our *body-egos* are always originally identified with the androgynous female mother-figure—that will hopefully give birth to a new foundational, truly personal ego. The fact that she is portrayed as a whore shows, on the one hand, that the patient is overcoming his life-long paranoia. He has always been afraid of being fucked, so to speak. On the other hand, it shows the direction the next stage of therapy will have to take: arrive at a distinction between sexual *Eros,* and the nonerotic forms of spiritual love, which the Greeks term *Agape*—charitable love, and *Philia*—brotherly love.

Let me give an example of a woman patient. She dreamed of entering a ladies' room and looking into a mirror. But she was disturbed by a filmy coating over the mirror surface which she knew to be a woman's "come," ejaculation of sperm. It was clear to me that this patient's unconscious mind finally picked up what was obvious to me from the beginning of treatment, that she was spiritually raped by her "macho-mother." For the baby's first mirror is the mother's facial expressiveness. This dream is a beautiful portrayal of the Greek conception of mind as *logos spermatikos,* in this case the penetrating phallic quality of the mother's look—the kind of formative experience that Freud saw as happening only with the father.

EMS: From what I gather, infancy is almost an effective dream in itself.

HE: It depends on the Kleinian. Someone like Donald Meltzer takes dreams very seriously.

EMS: But most of the recent Kleinian thinkers, some not even therapists, such as Norman Brown (1959), take it to the life-and-death struggle of the individual and the collective.

You see the infant getting discovered in the adult. As you spoke I tried to speculate how the development of moral character and its universal spiritual qualities begins to show in infancy.

HE: This is where what Kleinians call the infant's guilt comes in. Every baby feels guilty—inevitably feels guilty in the course of relations with the mother.

EMS: Or the moral imperative in terms of *Jahweh*—the judgmental God? But does infancy also bring out an immediate feeling of a kind of grand pantheism?

HE: I would say this. It's generally taken for granted in psychoanalysis that the first non-self, the first other, is the mother. Or if not the mother, what's called a part object, the breast. Now if you examine the baby's experience closely, without ideological preconceptions, you see that this is nonsense. The first non-self or other is an all-encompassing, spontaneously animated cosmos, centered in the mother's face as the focal point of interest. We see a little baby in a crib. We say: Here's the baby, there's the mother, there's the floor, the ceiling, the smells coming from the kitchen, light coming through the window—we distinguish a hundred different things. But when that baby first arrives at self-awareness, at a sense of Selfhood, it can't make such distinctions. The non-self is an all-encompassing kaleidoscopic surround. It gets dark, it gets light, there are noises and smells; and this first other I call the *Primordial Other*. And it's fundamentally the uniquely Hebrew conception of God. That's the great originality of the Hebraic tradition, to base all human experience on the original formative human experience of Selfhood, before the baby is aware of mother, or of mother's breast, as distinct bounded entities in space. It then comes into the spacial world of bounded material objects in space, after the sixth month, as "a child of God."

EMS: Is it a matter of which god we're talking about: the Hebraic God, a grand all-in-all, or a kind of cosmic essence?

HE: It's only the Hebraic God because by definition any bounded image is automatically an idol. And if you give it a name, thereby delimiting it, it's an idol. This distinguishes the original experience of the Primordial Other from its later vicissitudes, which I'll go into.

EMS: At the heart of Abraham's sojourn—and later in the formulation of the First Commandment—was the condemnation of idolatry. In contrast, inherent in the thinking of Jung is a kind of gnosticism. There is however, in Jungian thinking, a keen reverence for a *participation mystique*.

HE: Yes. Jungians have a respect for the mystical-religious dimension, but see it only in a way that corresponds to the baby's later development, after the onset of Melanie Klein's depressive position, which is after the eighth month of life.

EMS: Is this Melanie Klein or Henry Elkin? Who starts with the notion of primordial terror?

HE: We both start with the baby's terror and go on to the baby's guilt. But the terror, implied in Klein's paranoid-schizoid position, which she put in the third month, can't possibly be toward mother. It is rather the baby's overwhelming, reverential *awe* toward the Primordial Other, and culminates in what Erikson (1977) calls *basic trust* by the sixth month when the child first enters upon the material and spacial world of distinctly bounded entities like "Mother."

EMS: Is it the baby's guilt which Melanie Klein (1949) sees as the cornerstone of the depressive position?

HE: The baby's guilt for having injured the mother which Klein accounts for by her teacher Ferenczi's concept of infantile omnipotence, which accords with Freud's concept of primary narcissism, now discredited by both the object-relations approach and empirical research on infantile behavior.

To the baby at 8 months of age, the mother is like a 20-story skyscraper. The baby realizes that it is utterly puny, helpless, and dependent for its life on her ministrations. Why does it feel guilty for having injured this mother? Infantile omnipotence can only be accounted for by the baby's being in union, co-union, or communion, with the Primordial Other. This, moreover, is the true foundation of narcissism, in both its positive and negative aspects, as Heinz Kohut (1977) sees it.

EMS: Jung implies that Self is indistinguishable from the experience of God, or Divine Being. Since babies make no initial distinctions between object and subject, in the experience of the infant all disparate elements exist in effective union.

HE: Yes, but only in what I call the primordial stage of life, before the baby's conscious entry upon the material, spacial world in the sixth month of age.

EMS: Do we not then get to the need to individuate? I gather you think this is a terribly difficult task accomplished within that first year of life.

HE: It's only the foundations that are laid down at this time.

EMS: How so?

HE: After 8 months of age—the sixth to eighth month I call the *transi-*

122

tional stage—Ferenczi's infantile omnipotence based on the infant's mental-spiritual communion with the Primordial Other, a *No-thing,* still applies. Thus when the baby sees the mother as unhappy, it feels guilty. "I must have bit too hard. I damaged her with my teeth. That's why she looks so sad." We're dealing with the stage of oral aggression. Then, in the same period, the baby gets enraged—it's hungry, and has a temper tantrum. What does the mother do? She cuddles and caresses the baby. Thereby she erotically seduces it. Ferenczi saw this clearly, and recognized it as the foundation of all hypnotism and suggestibility. Eventually it becomes a kind of a mutual seduction. This happens in all normal healthy development. Every normal baby has somehow gotten into a pattern of mutual seduction with mama. An extreme example that I sometimes use in teaching: The baby says, "Ah, to make Mother happy. I'll behave like a zombie." This begins the normal split between what I call the mental, or more accurately, the *Transcendental-Ego,* and the *Body-Ego* whose dynamisms are thereby inhibited and repressed. The Transcendental-Ego, hitherto in communion with the Primordial Other, thus becomes the seductive and manipulative mind of what I call the "foxy baby," which replaces the "baby killer"; that is, violent aggression gets mentally-spiritually sublimated. But it is then normally lost to consciousness, to become what I call the *schizoid ego.* This operates in a hidden chamber in the back of the mind that says, "Ain't I smart! I know that if I behave like a zombie I'll make mother happy." The foxy baby and the schizoid ego are the experiential foundation for the age-old concept of original sin. Somewhere in the back of the minds of all who join up in collective movements or who take up prevailing fads there's the hidden thought, "Ain't I smart. I know how to make myself popular or socially acceptable." The hidden schizoid ego usually shows up in dreams where the dreamer is amazed to discover a hitherto concealed room or closet in his or her own home. Be it noted that the schizoid ego is a normal, inevitable aspect of human life.

EMS: So the development of shadow remains a lack of something. Perhaps the inability to maintain a seamless web of self. Is it the fragmentation of the self which ultimately results in individuation? Or is the Jungian notion of individuation literally a donation of the self from the broad collective? In the mythos of Genesis, the human was expelled from the Garden because of offensiveness to God. Adam and Eve had presumed a sense of Self.

HE: For the Kleinians the motive force for normal socialization is "reparation for guilt." Winnicott extends this to "capacity for concern." Jung's concept of individuation as the goal of therapy drew me to him from the start. For he implied by this concept the psychic liberation from parental figures. In my Freud-Jung synthesis, therapy has to go beyond reparation for guilt, which still implies subjection to parentally derived *superegos.* Insofar as the ego is grounded on communion with the Primordial Other, St. Augustine's dictum applies: "Love and do what thou wilt." Jung's archetypal shadow, to the effect of "love and hate, and then do what thou wilt," may well promote social effectiveness in the world, as I said, but in sharp contrast to the "freedom of the children of God."

It's on this score that I've had to go back to Freud. Liberation from subjection to parental superegos can be achieved only by resolving the oedipal complex, but on a far deeper level than Freud could ever envisage, on an ontological or what I familiarly call the Yin-Yang level as prefigured in Taoism. This reflects the baby's clear-cut distinction between the unbounded, nonmaterial "Father in Heaven" and "Mother Earth." They then get confused in Melanie Klein's depressive position after the eighth month. For the mental seduction that then occurs between mother and baby leads to replacing "Father in Heaven" by the experience of the all-powerful "Great Cosmic Mother." The mind of the original "foxy baby" that learned to seduce and manipulate mother, in becoming the hidden schizoid ego, is lost to consciousness. The baby remains aware only of the mother's overwhelming power on which it is totally dependent. Thus she becomes the *Great Mother Goddess.* This is the core of Jung's own pathology. Blind to his own schizoid ego, he attributed mental-spiritual *transcendence,* that which distinguishes the human from the animal, to the biologically inherited collective unconscious, when it is in fact the experiential foundation of individual *human* being. We don't call animals "persons," for they have no mental-spiritual transcendence. What I call the Transcendental-Ego is clearly shown in dreams—as when the dreamer is high up, on top of a mountain or building, surveying what lies beneath on earth. When the dream is flying through the air, it's the Transcendental-Ego but split off from Body-Ego.

EMS: How would this contrast with other views of a derivative theory? The fact that the infant emerges as a person from this whole primordial scene indicates that the baby becomes this to some degree, as an other. This then is true parenting—the primordial ground of being.

HE: True parenting?

EMS: Yes. It's where you have some justification for a theistic notion inasmuch as primordial parenting is not with the visible parents. We're all part of that collective.

HE: As human beings, our parents function more or less as mediators, mediators to the original "God-given Self."

EMS: In terms of contrast, we have both a Jungian and a Winnicottian notion of good-enough mothering as a prelude to individuation.

HE: Good-enough mothering is mothering whereby the mother functions to a marked degree as a mediatrice to the child's autonomous God-given Selfhood. For example, the mother and child play together: Mother puts food in the baby's mouth, and baby puts food in the mother's mouth. They are here equals in the "presence of God."

EMS: True birth, then, takes place on behalf of the whole cosmos. Mother fulfills a universal task.

I get no sense of a drive theory in Jung. In Freud you have a libidinal drive theory. In (Jacques) Lacanian terms, it's no so much drive, but *desire* (Lacan, 1977). Desire resonates with the mother's engagement. There are many many bridges indeed.

You do use the notion of the archetypes in your therapy, do you?

HE: When I do, I say, "what Jungians call archetypes," to avoid the Jungian sense of biological or racial inheritance. I think of them as universal biologically grounded forms of thought or behavior.

EMS: The reason I ask is because you speak of a need to avoid idolatry. Do the archetypes become idols?

HE: Idols to me are superego images, inevitable in every society. All human society is grounded on some form of ancestor worship. We don't, like animals, simply disregard human corpses. The dead bodies of family, clan, and tribal members have always evoked mystical-religious awe, institutionalized in some form of funeral service. Thus in the face of death, and in the conscious awareness of death, human beings, by definition so to speak, have always been concerned with the meaning of life. Hence mythology. We all lead our lives in terms of some mythology, conscious or unconscious. Jung's turn to the systematic study of mythology goes along with his dream interpretation, to discover the hidden mythology that guides the dreamer's actual life.

It's only in this context of inevitable idolatry, of superego and ego-ideal images rooted in the earliest experience of parents and siblings, that the extraordinary novelty of the Hebraic spirit can be properly grasped. The conflict with idolatry brings a permanent tension in the psyche which, in conjunction with Greek philosophy and Roman law, has given rise to the extreme dynamism of Western, and now all human, history. In simple realistic fact the Hebrew "God" has proved to be the "Lord of History," and in view of current space exploration, even of Cosmic History.

EMS: In another vein, do you see true individuation as ultimate integrity? In the same sense, does the development of conscience equal the integration of being? Together they forge the superego, which is not necessarily one with conscience. I tend to see the superego as a thou—developing to a representation of the beginning of the godhead. As you talk, I begin to piece together what true individuation means as primordial and personal development, because it calls forth the ability to respond to life in an integrated way.

HE: It's the Judeo-Christian experience of one's self as a "child of God" that explains the function of the *King* and *Queen* images in Jung's (1955/1963) studies of alchemical texts. They reflect the autonomy, the sovereignty of personal Selfhood. And whatever the tensions and conflicts of Western history, actual kings and queens, moveover, like the Chinese emperors, functioned like "good-enough mothers" or "good-enough fathers"; that is, they functioned ceremonially, ritually, in acknowledging their subordination to "God in heaven." The image of medieval kings, like Popes, washing the feet of 12 beggars on Good Friday, is a most powerful image. The contradiction between the ideal and the concrete actual reality of worldly authority gave rise to the Reformation, of course, and to all that followed. It's not for us to judge. In truth, I'm tempted to think of Chinese civilization as far more preferable. The fact that the warrior class was always subordinate to the Confucian intellectual bureaucracy gave Chinese history an enviable stability over more than 2,000 years. The dynamism of Western history must simply be accepted on faith, for better or worse. Jung always admonished his followers to avoid trying to become like Orientals.

EMS: Moving ahead, I was thinking of the three significant revolutions that Freud was said to have referred to. The Copernican revolution ushered in the moment in which humans no longer saw themselves as the center of the universe. Then the Darwinian revolution did its best to incarnate the collective. The third—the psychoanalytic revolution—displaced consciousness, seeing it as not really in charge of anything. From what you talked about, there is some need of redoing this schema. Indeed, each of us is experientially at the center in order to be able to encompass the primordial awe. Without the stargazer there is no universe.

HE: Freud is here saying, "It's me, Sigmund Freud, who's bringing about the third great revolution." I agree with him. Jung does too, implicitly. Freud's great revolutionary contribution was to apply the Hebraic conception of the meaningful course of history to the individual's actual life experience. The fact that he did this by way of extending the thought patterns of 19th-century natural history, Lyell's geology, and especially Darwin's biology, over into the human realm makes for the inherent contradictions in Freudian theory. As a good Darwinian, he had to begin with his theory of drives. However much his subsequent thought radically deviated from it, he affirmed it to the very end, stultifying the development of psychoanalysis. As I see it, this was the final outcome of Freud's upholding his sexual determinism over against what he saw as Jung's mystifications. Don't overlook the fact, however, that Jung was a far more thoroughgoing Darwinian in his belief in the racial unconscious that he invariably applied in clinical practice, and in his conviction that each individual animal and plant also had their divinely grounded Selves—good 19th-century nature mysticism.

EMS: But isn't there a deep kinship with nature that Freud overlooks?

HE: Yes, to be sure, because of Freud's obsessions with sexuality. Jung's recognition of this kinship compensated for Freud's blindness. But Jung perceived this kinship only in its secondary form, with relation to the Great Mother Goddess. Its initial form arose with the emergence of the *Primordial Self* in communion with the all-encompassing Primordial Other. Referring to "God" as "Father in Heaven," whether in the Judeo-Christian tradition or in the Chinese tradition, was never taken literally. It's only a verbal metaphor to offset the danger of blind fusion with and enslavement to Mother, or Mother Nature.

This is why I see the goal of therapy as the resolution of the oedipal, but on a far deeper level than Freud ever envisaged. Moreover, it's precisely here that Jung can be of great help. Whereas Freud only saw bisexuality as linked to perversion, Jung saw it as the foundation of the individuation process. One great truth I picked up in Zurich is that to achieve proper masculinity a man must develop his "feminine" side; and that a woman, correspondingly, to achieve proper femininity, must develop her "masculine" side. But this is only valid within the larger context provided by the goal of resolving the oedipal. Jung pretty much restricted his view to the introverted psychic life, separate from the actuality of social existence. Thus Jungian psychology fostered a deep psychic split, not unlike that of pietistic sects, Quakers, and Christian Scientists. It is this schizoid split that has given rise to the sharp divergences that have ensued in Jungian psychology. On the one hand there is the assimilation of Kleinian and other "object relations" theory, the

127

direction I have taken. On the other hand, there is widespread Jungian support of ideological feminism by promoting the woman's overly facile identification with the Great Mother Goddess. This rules out any resolution of the oedipal.

Let's first look at the man's situation. The key point I want to make is that his femininity must be developed within the context of his psychobiological maleness. This is where the problem of psychic "homosexuality" arises, the problem in Freud's relation to Wilhelm Fliess that first gave rise to psychoanalysis, and then in Freud and Jung's relation to one another that determined its subsequent history. The recent superb book by Joyce McDougall (1985), a London-trained Kleinian practicing in Paris for 30 years, clearly shows how the problem of homosexuality arises through unresolved mother-baby relations. It is only by achieving a deep sense of *personal identity,* grounded in the primordial stage of life when the baby is still only a "child of God," that the problem of *sexual identity* can be properly resolved.

Here is where a clear-cut distinction between the *Body-Ego* and the *Transcendental-Ego,* which occurs following Melanie Klein's depressive position in the eighth month, is imperative. The Body-Ego, the seat of Freud's libido and aggression, remains forever grounded on identification with the original caretaking mother, experienced as androgynous. One must never refer to the original mother as feminine! Confusion regarding sexual identity reflects the failure to distinguish psychobiological *maleness* and *femaleness* from mental-spiritual *masculinity*—aggressiveness or assertiveness, and *femininity*—mental-spiritual receptivity. The original caretaking mother with whom the child's Body-Ego remains forever identified is *female.*

A striking case in point is the image of the football player. His immense broad shoulders and chest, scarcely visible face, absolute self-assurance both at rest and when breaking out into sudden powerful movements focused upon retaining possession of the precious ball—an image reflecting the baby's experience of its tiny, helpless physical self—clearly recaptures the image of Mother as female. In a world that tends to restrict the conception of masculinity to Body-Ego terms, the man's femininity, his erotically grounded receptivity, will tend to be restricted to team solidarity and "buddy" relationships.

Let's get to the woman's situation. The Great Mother Goddess, seen as an image of ultimate cosmic Divinity and functioning in support of the woman's ego-ideal, is not an image of her natural femaleness. For it tends to rule out that aspect of femaleness that passively surrenders to biological maleness. At this point another distinction is imperative, one I regard as Lacan's (1977) great contribution: that between the mental-spiritual phallus and the anatomical penis. The incipient danger in the woman's acquiring phallic mental-spiritual power is the temptation to direct her female tendencies toward seductive manipulative goals. This is the very essence of narcissism, which can't surrender to anything. Hasn't this become a widespread ego-ideal? Namely, the Cosmo girl who "has everything." On the other hand, the truly creative woman, in whatever field, doesn't use her phallic power in this way and is not to be found among the doctrinaire feminists.

EMS: What you say moves through the notion of sexual equality to the phenomenon of sexual identity.

HE: Husbands being the prime caretaker of children in the home, and especially of babies, is perhaps the most thoroughgoing perversion of nature to be found in all human history. But fathers have played a most important formative role, at least in all higher civilizations. Perceived by the small child far less by touch or smell—surely not by taste!—than by sight and hearing, and as regularly going off and returning from the "infinite horizon," the *initial* Father image became a fitting object on which the small child transferred its experience of the Primordial Other. Freud got it backwards, in reverse order, by calling "God" a father projection.

EMS: Freud's patriarchy, male chauvinism?

HE: Yes, Freud's playing the role of patriarch was his form of therapeutic psychopathy. But doctrinaire feminism, in its attacks on patriarchy, has blurred over the radical distinction between Hebraic and Roman patriarchy, for example. The unique feature of Hebrew patriarchy is that the original patriarchs, Abraham, Isaac, and Jacob, were always masterminded, in effect, by the *de facto* matriarchs, Sarah, Rebecca, and Rachel. Thereby in the course of subsequent history the Hebraic man came to assimilate within the context of his given maleness the incipient feminine spirituality of the woman.

EMS: How to bring it all together?

HE: My aim is to help bring about a reconciliation of Freud and Jung through a proper synthesis of their great pioneering contributions. Thus we may hopefully recuperate the fundamental psychological truth of Judeo-Christianity that determined the course of Western history, and bring it into harmonious and creative interaction with the deep wisdom of the Orient with regard to mind-body integration. Freud and Jung can be our mediators to the reconciliation of "Father in Heaven" and "Mother Earth" within ourselves.

REFERENCES

Brown, N. (1959). *Life against death: The psychoanalytic meaning of history.* Middletown, CT: Wesleyan University Press.

Erikson, E. H. (1977). *Identity and the life cycle.* New York: International Universities Press.

Jung, C. G. (1954). Answer to Job. In H. Read, H. Fordham, Adler, G. & McGuire, W. (Eds.) and R. F. C. Hull (Trans.), *The collected works of C. G. Jung* (Vol. 11, pp. 553-758). Princeton: Princeton University Press/Bollingen Series XX.

Jung, C. G. (1963). Mysterium coniunctionis. In H. Read, M. Fordham, & G. Adler (Eds.) and R. Hull (Trans.), *The collected works of C. G. Jung* (Vol. 14). New York: Pantheon/Bollingen Series XX. (Original work published 1955.)

Klein, M. (1949). *The psychoanalysis of children.* London: Hogarth Press.

Kohut, H. (1977). *The restoration of the self.* New York: International Universities Press.

Lacan, J. (1977). *Ecrits, A selection.* New York: Norton.

McDougall, J. (1985). *Theaters of the mind. Illusion and truth on the pyschoanalytic stage.* New York: Basic Books.

Meltzer, D. (1983). *Dream-life, A reexamination of psychoanalytical theory and technique.* Perthshire, Scotland: Clunie Press.

Segal, H. (1964). *Introduction to the work of Melanie Klein.* New York: Basic Books.

Spitz, R. (1965). *The first year of life.* New York: International Universities Press.

White, V. (1960). *Soul and psyche: An enquiry into the relationship of psychology and religion.* London: Collins.

Winnicott, D. W. (1965). *The maturational process and the facilitating environment.* New York: International Universities Press.

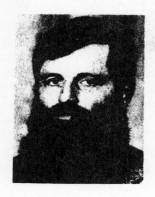

Eugene Taylor

C. G. Jung and the Boston Psychopathologists, 1902-1912*

Eugene Taylor is Associate in Psychiatry, Harvard Medical School, and Consultant in the History of Psychiatry at the Massachusetts General Hospital. He is the author of *William James on Exceptional Mental States* (New York, Scribner's, 1983).

10 Shattuck Street
Boston, Massachusetts 02115

From 1880 to 1920, Boston was the center of psychotherapeutic developments in the English-speaking world (Burnham, 1958, 1967; Hale, 1971; Gifford, 1978); and as recent investigation of this important period in Boston history has shown, long before Freud, there flourished a uniquely American dynamic psychology of the subconscious (Taylor, 1982a, 1982b, 1983, 1985a)—one that for various reasons embraced Jung earlier than Freud and, on a number of important points, resembled Jung's version of psychoanalysis more closely than Freud's. In fact, an examination of Jung's association with the psychotherapeutic practitioners of Boston allows us, I believe, to address a particularly vexing problem in the history of psychology and psychiatry, namely, the persistence of the stereotype that Jung was "nothing but" Freud's disciple. Indeed, I shall claim that the wider context of Jung's associations, before, during, and after his exchange with Freud, shows a consistency that allows Jung the privilege of being assessed in his own right, for the most part independent of any subservient historical debt to Freudian theory.

To do this, I would like to examine Jung's association with three of the Boston group: Adolf Meyer, Swiss psychiatrist who was pathologist at the Worcester State Hospital from 1896 to 1902, although it was a few years later, during his tenure as head of the New York State asylum system, that Meyer actually interacted with Jung; James Jackson Putnam, Professor of Diseases of the Nervous System at Harvard Medical School and main supporter of Freud's ideas in Boston after 1909, who nevertheless read and critiqued Jung avidly; and finally, William James, philosopher-psychologist at Harvard, the man who first introduced Breuer and Freud to the American psychological public in 1894 (Burnham, 1956; Ross, 1978), but whose interest in psychopathology, like Jung's, followed the

---

* This paper was originally presented for the History Division of the American Psychological Association in Los Angeles, California, August 26, 1985.

lines of Janet's studies in the so-called French Experimental Psychology of the Subconscious and Meyers and Gurney's work through the English Society for Psychical Research.

Jung and Meyer

Meyer, like Jung, had come from the Zurich school of psychiatry. Meyer had studied under the famous brain neuroanatomist, August Forel, who moved into psychiatry when he became head of the Burghölzli Asylum and transformed it into an internationally recognized hospital that was renowned for its scientific orientation. It was Egen Bleuler, Forel's student and Jung's teacher, who became head of the Burghölzli after Forel and guided Jung through his early medical career just at the turn of the century.

Meyer, who had taken his degree some 10 years earlier, had emigrated to the United States in 1891 and spent almost 5 years associated with the University of Chicago and the Kankakee State Hospital before being wooed to the Worcester State Hospital just outside Boston by G. Stanley Hall, President of nearby Clark University, and Edward Cowles, Superintendent of the McLean Hospital, who taught psychiatry at Harvard Medical School (Grob, 1966). Meyer remained at Worcester just long enough to test out various aspects of his psychobiosocial approach to the treatment of insanity before moving to New York in 1902 to take charge of the Pathological Institute there, which meant medical control of the state's asylum system. In his capacity as chief pathologist at the Worcester State Hospital, Meyer had regular contacts with Boston physicians in charge of other local asylums, and frequent interchanges with men such as James Jackson Putnam, E. W. Taylor, George Waterman, Isador Coriat, and William James, all of whom were involved in experimenting with the newest developments in psychotherapeutic treatment (Hale, 1971, 1978).

Meyer had been exposed to the introduction of Breuer and Freud's ideas into Boston through James and Putnam from the time of his arrival in 1896, but always within the context of other psychotherapeutic systems then in vogue, chiefly those of Janet, Prince, Sturgis, and Sidis. The attitude was eclectic, and Freud's ideas stood out no more than anyone else's, except those of Janet, who, in Boston as in Zurich, was given precedence for his discovery of the symbolic nature of hysteric symptoms, for Charcot's idea that the source of psychoneurotic symptoms can be found hidden in forgotten traumatic memories, and for his detailed patient histories. On the other hand, Freud was consistently presented as second author to Breuer, a practice which continued in Boston circles at least up to 1904 (Taylor, 1984, 1985).

By 1902, Meyer had moved to New York, and it was during this period that his relationship with Jung formally developed. He must have known of Jung's association experiments at the Burghölzli in 1904, and he certainly knew of them by 1906 through Morton Prince's Boston-based *Journal of Abnormal Psychology*. In addition, Meyer's staff in New York had early contacts with Jung. G. H. Kirby visited Jung in late 1906, and in early 1907, at Meyer's suggestion, the New York neurologist, Frederick Peterson, spent several weeks with Jung, resulting in two jointly authored papers on the psycho-galvanic reflex (Leys, 1985).

Meyer's correspondence with Jung then opened in July of 1907, and lasted until 1913. Their exchange was no doubt originally based on their mutual contempt for Kraepelinian nosology and, more important, on Meyer's sense that Jung's psychology was much like his own approach to mental illness, based on the pragmatism of William James and the functionalism of John Dewey.

Meyer went on to review both Freud and Jung frequently between 1905 and 1908, and according to Leys (1985), Jung's association experiments appear to have stimulated Meyer's engagement with Freud's theoretical writings. Meyer encouraged members of his staff to use the word-association test in their clinical work (Leys, 1985), while at the same time Meyer promoted the use of Freud's method of psychoanalysis (Hale, 1971).

While it is probably true that both Jung and Meyer showed a common appreciation for the hope held out by psychotherapeutic methods in treating the psychoses, and that Meyer and Jung shared a common appreciation for the experimental corroboration provided by the word-association test,[1] it is also probably true that as time went on, Meyer con-

---

1. Originally derived from the experimental methods of Wundt and Galton, the word-association test was first adapted to depth-psychology by Jung and Riklin as an objective measure of subconscious complexes. Jung withstood a number of criticisms of this method until the German psychologist, William Stern, claimed that the method was not objective, for the reason that Jung's subjects were untrained introspective observers and, without the proper expertise, were incapable of giving an accurate description of their inner sensations. According to Kerr (1985), it was as a result of this attack that Jung first publicly adopted Freud's theory of psychoanalysis, in late 1905, in order to justify his own interpretation. Freud, however, held the association method as foreign to psychoanalysis. In fact, the association test presented a significant threat to his clinical findings and the logic of his system, for the reason that it held the possibility of galvanizing scientific attention on methods of laboratory verification, slighting what Freud felt to be more important, namely, psychoanalytic procedures, which were verified by Freud's own clinical observations. Meanwhile, Jung's association experiment had been eagerly taken up by the Boston psychopathologists, such as Morton Prince, Isador Coriat, and Boris Sidis, precisely because it provided experimental verification for one element of their contemporary psychotherapeutic practice, flourishing, albeit desperate for any and all scientific credentials. In this vein, Jung's association method, Cannon's physiological work on the viscera and the emotions, and Pavlov's conditioning experiments were being incorporated into the Boston scene as early as 1904.

tributed in no small measure to the perception that Jung was Freud's disciple: first, because Meyer took much of his interpretation of Freud through Jung's writings before 1909, and then further associated the two together as a result of the Clark University Conference. Meyer also spoke at Clark, but attracted much less attention than Freud or Jung, partly because he lectured only once—on the difficult topic of psychotherapy with the insane. Indeed, American psychological history has perpetuated a stereotype of Freud and Jung at the Clark Conference that has left Meyer largely forgotten. Meyer, in his later life, expressed bitterness over this state of affairs, although he may have unwittingly helped to perpetuate it. His perceptions of Jung, we might say, were equivocal.

Immediately after the Clark Conference, for instance, Meyer opened correspondence with E. B. Titchener, another speaker at Clark, in an attempt to reconcile some of the great differences between experimental psychology and dynamic psychiatry that the Clark lectures had revealed (Leys, 1985). Titchener was a forceful advocate for Wundtian methods of laboratory science, but Meyer tried to argue favorably on the experimental foundation of depth-psychology, using Jung's association studies as proof. At the same time, however, following the Clark Conference, Meyer's close friend and eventual successor at the Pathological Institute in New York, August Hoch, went for an extended visit to Zurich, where he studied with Jung, underwent a brief period of treatment for depression, and became a strong supporter of Jung's version of psychoanalysis.

Jung must have had, even then, a charismatic appeal to the subconscious of his patients and colleagues, for shortly after he left America with Freud and Ferenczi, Meyer had a dream about him that was recorded and preserved, but never analyzed by Meyer (Leys, 1985). We also see Meyer taking up a defense of Jung's sexual interpretations against attacks by American physicians on several occasions. Thus, Meyer seems to have had connections with Jung independent of psychoanalysis *per se,* but also clearly associated with it.

Could it be, in this regard, that Meyer and his staff, by retailing Freud through Jung, were actually, and unwittingly, propounding more of Jung than of Freud? Several factors suggest that such an interpretation may be the case. First, Meyer knew Jung better than he knew Freud. Meyer and Jung had contact on many occasions, whereas Meyer had met Freud only twice, and had a chance to talk with him only once. Second, to be a psychoanalyst in America before 1909 meant that anyone doing therapy had read Freud or Jung and incorporated their ideas into patient practice. This was long before the requirement of analysis with Freud himself, a fate that both Meyer and Jung eventually escaped anyway, and also before the rise of the psychoanalytic organizations and institutions. Third, both

Jung and Meyer worked with the same population of patients, asylum inmates, who were much more difficult to treat psychotherapeutically than the office patients of Freud. And fourth, as Leys (1985) points out, Meyer played a major role in the desexualization of Freud's theories in America. Jung's interpretation of Freud's theory, history shows us, has had much the same effect.

Paradoxically, however, it was just when the break between Jung and Freud was imminent, bringing Jung much closer theoretically to Meyer, that the association between Jung and Meyer came to an end. Leys explains that Meyer saw the rift between Jung and Freud gaining international attention and this would have disastrous effects for Meyer's own plan to promote dynamic psychiatry within the conservative American medical profession. How could psychiatry gain acceptance, in other words, if there was no scientific, clinical, or methodological consensus within that field? He thought the Jung-Freud debate a very cheap and weak affair, which only proved his own belief in the superiority of American psychiatry, with its more collaborative spirit, and pragmatic emphasis on common sense, problem solving, and practical results (Leys, 1985).

Jung and Putnam

The relationship between Jung and James Jackson Putnam, Harvard's first professor of neurology and the first to introduce psychoanalysis into the Massachusetts General Hospital as early as 1904 (Taylor, 1984), is important for a number of reasons, not the least of which is the light it sheds on Jung's analysis of Fanny Bowditch, probably Jung's first great success after the muddled Spielrein affair.[2] Fanny Bowditch was the daughter of Henry Pickering Bowditch, first research professor of physiology at Harvard Medical School, Dean of the medical faculty from 1883 to 1894, and colleague of both William James and James Jackson Putnam in launching the so-called Boston School of Psychotherapy. Bowditch had suffered a stroke in 1906 and Fanny attended to his needs for the last 5 years of his life. Shortly after his death in early 1911, Fanny went into a severe depression, complained of feelings of unreality, and was plagued by thoughts of suicide. The Bowditch family approached James Jackson Putnam, then perceived as American medicine's most ardent disciple of Freud, but, quite surprisingly, Putnam recommended that Fanny travel to Europe in the fall of 1911 for an analysis with Jung. Immediately, she began to correspond with Putnam about each phase of the analysis, sometimes writing him 30-page letters, while Putnam returned with advice, criticism, and encouragement until 1916, when Fanny broke

2. For details of the Spielrein, Jung, Freud relationship, see Carotenuto (1980, 1984). For the relationship of Jung to his first patient see Goodheart (1985).

off with Jung and 2 years later married Johann Rudolph Katz, a Dutch psychiatrist.

While all but two of Fanny's letters to Putnam have escaped preservation, some 22 letters of Putnam's in return are on deposit at the Countway Library of Medicine. These letters give us some clues as to the course of therapy and also provide us with a good picture of Putnam's changing perception of Jung, as well as the basis of Putnam's faith in him.

First, we see that Fanny's symptoms in the opening months of analysis continued and were evidently not helped by her difficulty in adjusting to Jung himself. Learning some of the details, Putnam (December 1, 1912) wrote:

> It is a fault in Dr. Jung that he is too self-assertive, lacking in some kind of needful imagination. He is indeed a strong but vain person who does much good, but also tends to crush a patient. He is to be learned from, but not followed too implicitly.

That personal development—a process he would later call individuation—was a major goal of Jung's therapeutic strategy is suggested even at this early date by a number of Putnam's letters. On August 13, 1912, for instance, Putnam wrote:

> The religious side of the matter, properly understood, is worth a vast deal in my opinion and though it, I believe, is not Dr. Jung's, I consider him as religious without realizing it. He is a "constructive idealist" to some extent.

And some months later, Putnam (December 9, 1912) wrote:

> I am going to write one of those philosophical papers of which I am so fond and so few other people care for, in which I hope to show that Dr. Jung's widened conception of the "libido" can be still further widened.

While the following year he was still trying to fathom Jung's religious orientation. He wrote on March 7, 1913:

> I am very curious about what Dr. Jung's religious views may be, and when you are to return, I want you to tell me all about them. His father, as of course you know, was a clergyman. But he broke off from that stem, and I assumed, after hearing what he told me at . . . [a recent congress] that he had no beliefs.

Actually, independent of Fanny's letters, Putnam and Jung had their own communications during this period. Putnam saw Jung, even if briefly, on several of his trips to America, and they were constantly exchanging papers by mail, critiquing each other in detail. Putnam evidently sensed more of the religious element in Fanny's treatment, however, than he got from Jung's publications. Putnam did comment to Fanny at one point on public reaction to Jung's work, obviously sympathizing now with Jung. On October 12, 1912, he wrote:

> I suppose it is not to be wondered at that your nice aunt, who is evidently pretty fixed in her ideas, should think Dr. Jung's ideas strange and reprehensible.
> You know, I imagine that even the majority of Drs. are very much "down" on the whole business—which means, of course, that (without being aware of it) they neglect their own patients.

Suggested here, in other words, is not Jung's support of Freud's ideas on psychoanalysis, but Jung's general appreciation of the importance of dynamic, subconscious factors and also the public and professional misunderstanding of the personal religious quest as an integral part of psychotherapy. Freud, as we know, opposed injecting the religious element into psychoanalysis, but encouraged Putnam to write about it anyway. Meanwhile, it was precisely on this question that Putnam and Jung were probably in closest agreement.

What signs there are in the Fanny Bowditch Katz papers at Harvard give us a general indication of the methods employed in Jung's therapy. These included having patients attend lectures and seminars given by Jung, in addition to individual therapy, which included the cultivation of the patient's powers of fantasy, the use of artistic productions to reveal hidden unconscious symbolism, in addition to the revelation through various means of unconscious complexes.

Most significant, however, was the successful manner in which Jung dealt with the transference. When the first signs of Fanny's bitterness, anger, and hostility became directed toward Jung, he employed the use of a female analyst, Maria Moltzer, in 1912. Moltzer kept in close contact with Fanny throughout the course of the therapy with Jung, interpreting, consoling, helping her to work through her feelings about Jung and to realize they were based on repressed parental problems. In fact, as a co-analyst, she probably conducted most of the therapy. When Fanny broke off the analysis with Jung in 1916, Moltzer kept up her therapeutic exchange and saw Fanny successfully through the 2 years that elapsed before her marriage to Katz in 1918.

The concept of the archetype appears as an interpretive dimension in their exchange, and was part of the language that Fanny used to describe "a death of the old personality," which occurred just before she ended her analysis with Jung. In June, 1916, she wrote:

> The thought came to me that in breaking the transference, which meant the tearing asunder of the bonds which had held me all my life—bonds which had kept me bound to the great-mother principle, as a child is bound to the mother, I must use all the strength in my personality, give all I have—and above all make it beautiful. (Katz, 1916)

She then described "a fantasy which needed to be lived," full of images that were to become for her, "the guardian of my roses and a symbol of new strength, of a new life, born of sacrifice and death" (Katz, 1916). We see here, in other words, the emergence of the rebirth motif that was to become a common part of Jung's psychology later on.

The composite picture, then, was that Jung handled the transference by using Moltzer to help the patient; meanwhile, Fanny was getting strong and constant support from Putnam by mail, since he was privy to all the intimate details of the analysis. In the beginning, Putnam's letters show how he gives a measure of support to her negative accounts of Jung. As the first 2 years pass, with both Jung and Moltzer helping her, she reaches a crisis point in the therapy and must return to America for a brief break, during which time her distortions of Jung to Putnam reach their height. On her return to Zurich, the first months of her continuing analysis bring her the emotional realization of the transference, which she responds to with exaggerated feelings of shame and guilt, confessing all to both Putnam and Jung. The next 3 years are spent in a beneficial but painful analysis of her family relationships and a search for her inner archetypal symbols. The result was the perceived death of her old personality; her break with Jung; followed 2 years later, with Moltzer's help, by Fanny's marriage. By then Putnam was writing Fanny to congratulate himself for having suggested Jung.

It is worth noting the progress Jung had made on an understanding of the transference since his analysis with Spielrein. At a time when Jung had turned to Freud for help in 1905, Freud's own understanding of the dynamics of the transference relationship were not yet completely formed. Thereafter, as if both had learned their lesson, Freud more clearly enunciated the transference theory as we know it today, while finally, at the Fordham lectures in 1912, which marked Jung's break with Freud, Jung himself gave a similar description of how to use the transference successfully in therapy. One could even say in this regard that an incomplete understanding of the transference was what plagued Jung and Freud the most in their own relationship, and it was not until the split between them that they came to fully understand it in the lives of their patients.

As for Jung's relation to Putnam, their common interest in the implications of personal, spiritual experience as a part of successful psychotherapy seems to be the key in understanding their relationship. Putnam, we know, was perceived in America as an arch Freudian, but he was never accepted as such within Freud's inner circle; and as to his relation with Freud, we know that Putnam held out for the inclusion of teleologic goals of personal meaning in psychoanalytic therapy—a philosophy for psychoanalysis, Putnam had called it. This meant that despite Putnam's early view of Jung as "too cosmic," it is clear that Jung's claim to an ethical and religious foundation for his psychology allied him much more with the intuitive and moral psychologies of character formation found in New England medical psychotherapy than with the theory of sublimated repression for purely social ends propounded by the Freudians.

Jung has left us with his assessment of Putnam, full of praise and gratitude. In the German edition of *Memories, Dreams, and Reflections,* not included in the English translations, Jung cited Putnam for his "unflapping desire for objectivity," his "open-mindedness," and his "readiness to give credit." Above all, Jung said, during the stormy period of separation with Freud, it was Putnam who pointed out that the general hostility to Freud's ideas was directed not only against the disreputable sexual theory, but against the point of view stressing the unconscious in general—that in fact the resistance was really to the unconscious, making the situation thoroughly complicated and obscure (cited in Taylor, 1980, p. 162).

Jung and James

William James must have had knowledge of Jung's work prior to their first and only meeting at the Clark Conference in 1909, again probably through Morton Prince's *Journal of Abnormal Psychology,* which carried articles by Jung or reviews of his work in nearly every issue beginning in 1906. Or, James could have come to know of Jung through August Forel and Theodore Flournoy, Boston's connections to the latest developments in Swiss psychiatry. Or, James could have heard of Jung through Janet, a friend and correspondent of James's, with whom Jung had studied during the winter of 1902-03.

In any event, Jung's meeting with James took place in G. Stanley Hall's house, with Freud, Hall, and a few others present. During dinner, Hall derided James's interest in psychical research, saying that James would arrive soon to talk about his most recent investigations of the medium, Mrs. Lenora Piper. When James appeared, he jokingly played on Hall's obsession with soliciting financial donations for Clark, which Hall brought up constantly to everyone, by reaching into his pocket for the Piper papers, but pulling out instead, a wad of dollar bills, much to everyone's amusement. Jung and James were given the opportunity to talk

139

alone for an hour, and Jung recounted that the subject of their conversation focused solely on their mutual interest in psychical research.[3]

We have James's annotated copy of Jung's dissertation, *On the Psychology and Pathology of So-Called Occult Phenomena* (Jung, 1902), which in all likelihood Jung gave to James at the time of their meeting. As was so characteristic of James with much of his reading, he apparently skipped the theoretical part of Jung's dissertation and, if his marginal marks tell the true story, read only the details of the case study.

James, Jung said, made a profound and lasting impression. James was distinguished, pleasant, quite natural, and without affectation or pomposity, and he spoke to Jung, some 30 years his junior, as an equal. Jung later wrote of James, saying, "Aside from Flournoy, he was the only outstanding mind with whom I could conduct an uncomplicated conversation" (cited in Taylor, 1980, p. 161).

By Jung's own account, however, a greater influence came about through Jung's reading of James's publishing writings. It was to James's *Pragmatism* that Jung turned in 1912 for philosophical justification over the break with Freud. It was to James that Jung turned for the philosophical contribution to the problem of psychological types. In an essay devoted to James and included in *Psychological Types,* Jung (1921) in particular, lauded James's formulations of inwardly versus outwardly directed personalities, as these ideas first appeared in James's (1890) *Principles of Psychology,* and then were developed in more mature form in James's (1907) *Pragmatism.*

---

3. Jung's interest in the occult at once divided him from Freud and more closely allied him with the Boston psychopathologists. Freud had taken up the topic on several occasions (Jones, 1957). It was a topic, however, he said that "perplexed him to distraction." He tended to interpret chance events along the lines of his personal superstitions, calling such occurrences telepathy. He was somewhat piqued that public opinion should show so many instinctive prepossessions against psychoanalysis, while the occult should so often be met half-way by powerful and mysterious sympathies. Freud said that his telepathic hypothesis was alien to psychoanalysis and could be explained on the basis of unconscious projection. On the other hand, he said he believed in telepathy, but could not personally explain it. He considered this paradox when revising *The Interpretation of Dreams* for the Collected Edition, saying "when anyone adduces my fall into sin, just answer him calmly that conversion to telepathy is my private affair, like my Jewishness, my passion for smoking, and many other things" (Jones 1953, pp. 395-396). Jung took up the problem of occult phenomena as the subject of his medical dissertation before he had ever met Freud, and through it he familiarized himself with a wide range of psychiatric literature then current. He continually differed with Freud over psychic events, believing himself capable of eliciting the phenomena, even in Freud's presence. Indeed, the occult for Jung was not a peripheral problem beyond science, but rather at the very heart of his psychology, for the psychic dimension of personality represented not the merely diabolical element within each one of us, but also unconscious creative ferment—the personality in transition, not for mere social adaptation, but for the forging of character—the achievement of the unique spiritual destiny of each individual.

Jung was also attracted to James's ideas on the ultra-marginal zone, or fringe of consciousness; the nature of the subliminal, following the work of F. W. H. Meyers; and James's conception of consciousness and the subconscious as a total region of different "fields" of possible awareness. Indeed, James's 1896 Lowell lectures on *Exceptional Mental States* accurately reflect the context of Jung's own exposure to and identification with such problems in psychology before 1902 (Taylor, 1983). James and Jung also held common attitudes about the limitations of contemporary science. Scientists, both agreed, had a common penchant for reducing everything of meaning and value to a "nothing but" philosophy. Finally, it was Jung's opportunity at the Harvard Tercentennary in 1936, when he received the L.L.D. degree, to praise James's psychological and pragmatic philosophy, which, he said, on more than one occasion had been his guide. There Jung also said of James, "It was his far-reaching mind which made me realize that the horizons of human psychology widen into the immeasurable" (cited in Taylor, 1980, p. 166).

Conclusion

Was Jung, then, a disciple of Freud's? At the most intense points of their relationship, as revealed in the recently published Freud-Jung correspondence (McGuire, 1974; Decker, 1980; Wollman, 1985), the water was so muddied that the roles of master-pupil, father-son, and moral versus immoral rival, were constantly being exaggerated or juxtaposed. Both obviously needed each other for their individual advancement. Freud never heard anything new at the end of their relationship that he had not already heard from the beginning (Stepansky, 1976). He needed Jung, however, both for the intellectual stimulation he lacked from within his own circle, and for the prestige that Jung brought from the world of asylum psychiatry, particularly Jung's non-Jewish Swiss connections. For his part, Jung probably viewed Freud's work as the only viable field of endeavor within European psychology or psychiatry that would accommodate his own more radical and unorthodox views about the psyche. Paradoxically, Jung was at first perceived as the more tame of the two because of his experimental work, while Freud was discounted because of his lurid sexual theories. History has shown, however, that by the 1930s, psychoanalysis began to gain a grudging admission into the psychological laboratories of the experimental psychologists (Rosenzweig, 1937, for instance) and into the medical curriculum of psychiatry (White, Wolfe, & Taylor, 1984), while Jung's psychology, with its archetypes, its mysticism, its alchemy, and its heavy emphasis on an inner language of spiritual transformation, *has never gained legitimate admission* into our universities and medical schools. In a sense, psychoanalysis has been admitted as the *de facto* depth-psychology, while Jung's more far-reaching formulations are summarily dismissed as "nothing but" a variant of Freud.

The great question remains, however, as to whether or not the scope of Jung's vision of the psyche and its potential for inner growth will ever become an integral part of present-day psychology. Is Jung now merely an historical anomaly, destined only to have been obscured by the apparent achievements of Freud's expertise as a political organizer for psychoanalysis? Were both men merely guilty of an overexaggerted sense of their own self-importance? Or is the scope and spirit of Jung's psychology perhaps a hint of what is yet to come? We may get a glimmer from Jung himself, when he enjoined his followers, the Jungian analysts, to create their own mythologies, not take up his own.

What may be called for, in other words, is a more radical change in our conception of human potential than the one inherent in the models and methods of what psychologists consider at present to be their legitimate domain—a psychology that is just as scientific and empirical, but now person-centered; far more transcendent; and, as Meyer, James, Putnam, and Jung have pleaded, perhaps far more relevant to the richness and variety of human experience.

REFERENCES

Burnham, J. C. (1956). The beginnings of psychoanalysis in the United States. *American Imago*, 65-68.

Burnham, J. C. (1958). *Psychoanalysis in American civilization before 1918.* Ann Arbor, MI: University Microfilms.

Burnham, J. C. (1967). *Psychoanalysis in American medicine, 1894-1918: Medicine, science, and culture. Psychological Issues Monograph 20, 5(4).*

Carotenuto, A. (1980). Sabina Spielrein and C. G. Jung: Some newly discovered documents bearing on psychotic transference, counter-transference, and the anima, *Spring*, 128-145.

Carotenuto, A. (1984). *A secret symmetry: Sabina Spielrein between Jung and Freud: The untold story of the woman who changed the early history of psychoanalysis.* New York: Pantheon.

Decker, H. S. (1980). A tangled skein: The Freud-Jung relationship. In E. R. Wallace & L. C. Pressley (Eds.), *Essays in the History of Psychiatry* (pp. 103-118). Columbia, SC: Wm. S. Hall Psychiatric Institute.

Gifford, E. G. (Ed.). (1978). *Psychoanalysis, psychotherapy, and the New England medical scene, 1894-1944.* New York: Science/History Pub.

Goodheart, W. B. (1984). C. G. Jung's first "patient": On the seminal emergence of Jung's thought. *Journal of Analytical Psychology, 29*(1), 1-34.

Grob, G. N. (1966). *The state and the mentally ill: A history of Worcester State Hospital in Massachusetts, 1830-1920.* Chapel Hill, NC: University of North Carolina Press.

Hale, N. G. (1971). *Freud and the Americans.* New York: Oxford University Press.

Hale, N. G. (1978). James Jackson Putnam and American neurology, 1877-1918. In E. G. Gifford (Ed.), *Psychoanalysis, psychotherapy, and the New England medical scene, 1894-1944* (pp. 149-154). New York: Science/History Pub.

James, W. (1890). *The principles of psychology* (Vol. 1-2). New York: Henry Holt.

James, W. (1907). *Pragmatism*. New York: Longmans, Green.

Jones, E. (1953). *The life and work of Sigmund Freud* (Vol. 3). New York: Basic Books.

Jung, C. G. (1902). *Zur Psychologie und Pathologie sogennter occulter Phänomene. Eine psychiatrische Studie.* Leipzig: Oswald Mutze. (William James's copy. James Papers. Houghton Library, Harvard University.)

Jung, C. G. (1921). *Psychologische Typen*. Zurich: Rascher.

Katz, F. B. (1916). Fantasy. Katz Papers. Harvard Medical Archives, Countway Library, Boston.

Kerr, J. (1985). *Spielrein, Freud, and Jung: The role of Sabina Spielrein in the founding of the International Psychoanalytic Movement.* Doctoral dissertation in preparation, New York University.

Leys, R. (1985). Meyer, Jung, and the limits of association. *Bulletin of the History of Medicine, 59*(3), 345-360.

McGuire, W. (Ed.). (1974). *The Freud/Jung letters: The correspondence between Sigmund Freud and Carl Jung.* Princeton: Princeton University Press.

Putnam, J. J. (1912-1913). Letters to Fanny Bowditch. Katz Papers. Harvard Medical Archives, Countway Library, Boston.

Ross, B. (1978). William James: A prime mover of the psychoanalytic movement in America. In E. G. Gifford (Ed.), *Psychoanalysis, psychotherapy, and the New England medical scene, 1894-1944* (pp. 10-23). New York: Science/History Pub.

Rosenzweig, S. (1937). The experimental study of psychoanalytic concepts. *Character and personality, 6*, 61-70.

Stepansky, P. (1976). The empiricist as rebel: Jung, Freud, and the burdens of discipleship. *Journal of the History of the Behavioral Science, 12*, 216-239.

Taylor, E. I. (1980). William James and C. G. Jung, *Spring*, 157-168.

Taylor, E. I. (1982a). William James on psychopathology: The 1896 Lowell lectures, *Harvard Library Bulletin, 30*(4), 455-479.

Taylor, E. I. (1982b). Louville Eugene Emerson: Psychotherapy, Harvard, and the early Boston scene, *Harvard Medical Alumni Bulletin*, 42-48.

Taylor, E. I. (1983). *William James on exceptional mental states: Reconstruction of 1896 Lowell lectures.* New York: Scribner's.

Taylor, E. I. (1984, May). *On the first use of psychoanalysis at the Massachusetts General Hospital, 1903-1905.* Paper presented at the annual meeting of the American Association for the History of Medicine, San Francisco, CA.

Taylor, E. I. (1985a, August 15). Psychotherapy, Harvard, and the American Society for Psychical Research, 1884-1889. *Proceedings of the 28th Annual Convention of the Parapsychological Association* (pp. 319-346). Medford, MA: Tufts University.

Taylor, E. I. (1958b). James Jackson Putnam's fateful meeting with Freud: The Clark University Conference of 1909. *VOICES: The Art and Science of Psychotherapy, 21*(1), 78-89.

White, B., Wolfe, R., & Taylor, E. I. (1984). *Stanley Cobb: A builder of the modern neurosciences* (pp. 197-218). Boston: Countway Library of Medicine/University of Virginia Press.

Wollman, N. J. (1984). Contrasts between Jung and Freud: The intertwining of life and theory. *Journal of Analytical Psychology, 29*(2), 171-186.

Acknowledgments are gratefully extended to Andrew Paskauskas, Institute for the History and Philosophy of Science and Technology, University of Toronto;

143

and to John Kerr, Department of Psychology, New York University, for extensive conversations and exchange of research materials; to Ruth Leys, Humanities Center, John Hopkins University, for graciously providing me with a prepublication draft of her Jung paper and her unpublished translation of the Meyer- Jung correspondence; to Roger Stoddard, Houghton Rare Manuscript Library, Harvard, for permission to refer to the William James Papers; to Richard Wolfe, Harvard Medical Archives, for access to the Fanny Bowditch Katz Papers; and to James Hillman for permission to paraphrase extensively from my James-Jung article in *Spring*.

Stanton Marlan

The Wandering Uterus:
Dream and the Pathologized Image

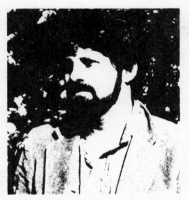

5400 Hobart Street
Pittsburgh, Pennsylvania 15217

Stanton Marlan, Ph.D., is a clinical psychologist, and a Jungian analyst in private practice. He received his doctorate from Duquesne University and is director of the Pittsburgh Center for Psychotherapy and Psychoanalysis. He is a senior analyst in the Inter-Regional Society of Jungian Analysts, and a member of the New York and International Societies for Analytical Psychology. His research interest in the last 4 years has been in an area of Archetypal Psychology. He resides in Pittsburgh with his wife Jan, also a psychologist, and has three children: Dawn, now at Bennington College; Tori, getting ready for college; and his son Brandon, 5, also researching archetypal figures.

> *For the soul to be struck to its imaginal*
> *depths . . . pathologizing fantasies are required.*
>
> JAMES HILLMAN
> *Revisioning Psychology*

Pathologized dream images are important to the soul. Acknowledging in the traditions of Freud and Jung the central value of the dream for analysis, Hillman (1975) goes on to emphasize those moments when dreams speak with pathologized images. Pathologizing, he states, "can take us out of blind immediacy," distorting our naturalistic view and moving us to a deeper reflection. The striking quality of such images breaks through our ordinary frames of reference, twisting, doubling, and compounding our consciousness and, as Hillman notes, reminding the soul of its mythical existence. For Hillman, pathologizing is mythmaking, and mythmaking is the way of soul.

To see the dream at the matrix of pathology and myth is to see both distortion and a new opening to the interior life. It is from this perspective that we can see not only how earlier dramas are currently being lived, but how the soul portends that ironic telos which Jung so well described. In the following I will present a dream of a young woman which contained pathologized images and which left me with a profound sense of soul.

Tara had been in a Jungian analysis in another state where she was also involved with a man who after 5 years cut off the relationship. She then made a decision to leave town and to pursue graduate education at a university near my practice. She started school but felt her life was not going well and she began to wonder if she had made the right choice in leaving. This concern led to our consultation. She felt it was important to be on her own, but she felt a deep wrenching inside that she did not understand. Being accustomed to the analytic situation, she presented the following dream.

> Out of her belly a white flat rubber band or cord is growing. It is wrapped around her head and she is pulled down into a depressed and fetal-like position. She asks her boyfriend to cut the cord and he does. There is pain and blood and she has a sense of a birth. She is now able to stand upright, and feels as if things might be OK, when all of a sudden her uterus falls out. She catches it in her hands and feels horrified.

In this dramatic and provoking dream, one intuitively gets the sense of a person undergoing a process of metamorphosis, of a movement in the soul from a depressed and embryonic state to a painful and bloody birth. Sticking with the images of the dream leads to a more precise and concrete understanding of the nature and meaning of Tara's suffering and further opens us to an expanded sense of her possibility. However, at the end of the dream we have an enigmatic image which at first seems to put this whole movement of individuation in question. One might imagine the dream in its linear and developmental sense, but this last image gives us pause and shakes us out of a simple sense of development, making us pay attention to the deeper adumbrations of the soul.

One could consider the dream as a response to her concern about having made the right move in leaving, but dreams are not usually oracular in a literal or objective sense; rather they allow us to see more deeply into what is going on below the questioning, into that matrix out of which the questioning arises.

As we began to talk about the dream, the feeling of being pulled down was prominent. She felt like an infant in a womb. Her struggle to extricate herself was countered by an elastic downward pull, drawing her head near to her belly as if there were something important to come close to and notice. Here one finds an image of her depression but, from a Jungian perspective, one begins to wonder about the intentionality of this symptom, of what it is she is being pulled down for. What is there at the belly that needs to be focused on and, further, what is this odd band or cord that seems to carry out this intention? Thinking about herself in the context of this first image spurred Tara's fantasy that this bond was like an umbilical cord and that she had been tied to her boyfriend in an infantile way. Like the cord itself, her relationship had become flat, and instead of feeling nourished, she felt drained, af if no vitality could pass between them.

146

Becoming conscious of these feelings led her to understand why in the dream she asked her boyfriend to cut the cord. In her conscious life she was not aware she wanted this severance or at least could not admit it to herself. To discover the congruence of her inner wish for separation with what actually happened gave her a sense of agency where she had felt none. She reflected on how it is that we can sometimes provoke others to carry out our wishes without being aware this is going on.

Our interpretation to this point has more or less been on what Jung would call the object level, that is, how the dream points to a relationship with the world, in this case, to her relationship with her boyfriend. But staying with the image rather than with the association suggests that what is binding and draws her down is what grows out of her own belly and wraps around her head, drawing it near. This observation leads to a more internalized sense of what is going on in the autonomous psyche and which may have been living itself out in her relationship with her boyfriend, but is intrinsically her own. This odd cord acts as if it has an intention of its own.

It is interesting to note that this cord image has been literalized in occult texts, particularly in the literature on astral projection, where it is seen as a manifestation of a subtle and vital process. It is said that emotion will increase its pull and that the astral body is very closely related to the dream body with which it is more or less identical (Carrington & Muldoon, 1929). It is provocative that the description of this cord is remarkably like that in Tara's dream. Many authorities hold that the "astral cord" adheres to the body at the solar plexus situated just behind the stomach which is where it emerged for Tara; and that while it is difficult to describe, it is like "an elastic cable, whitish grey in color."

From the naturalistic perspective what appears as a pathologized image is from the soul's view a connection to the subtle body of imagination and dream. This is not to say this cord is a literal object, but rather an archetypal image whose function is to connect us with ourselves, to our own deeper interiority.

From this perspective, one could say that the "figure" that the dream ego asks to cut the cord is her "boyfriend," it is also in another sense her inner masculine figure, or what Jung has called the animus. It is often the case that if a figure in a dream resembles an external one, the dream is interpreted in terms of that relationship. What I am suggesting is that the dream may simultaneously point to both the outer and inner level at the same moment; in fact, that it is rather an expression of the "in between" of objective and subjective, of boyfriend and animus, and as such is the matrix called psychic reality. Here the animus is the potential that could help release her from her depression, from her infantile belly-focused position. The simultaneity of both the importance of being close to her belly feelings and yet needing to free herself from them and to stand up is part of the complex doubling of the image.

It is the animus-boyfriend, her sharp incisive potential, that cuts through the flat, rubbery, and infantile depressive attachment, freeing her embryonic self through pain and blood for the birth of the upright self. Erwin Straus (1966) has stated that the upright posture distinguishes the human genus, and is the leitmotif in the formation of the human organism. To stand on one's own feet is also to be "upright," to stand for one's own convictions. This can be a terrifying and painful task involving separation, as it did for our dreamer.

Although on the outer level Tara had taken a stand, her soul was still moving in another and more dependent constellation. The psychological meaning of her uprightness still awaited the cutting of the inner cord. It is here that the connection of separation and being born, free to assume an upright posture, places her pain in another context, in the context of "birth." This somehow changes the quality of how her pain is experienced and gives it a new sense.

This upright movement brings with it a more horrific vision. Standing there, both in her new place in the world and within, her uterus spontaneously falls out. Had the dream ended before this image, it would have seemed complete and less perplexing, but the power of this pathologized image moves us to an even deeper dimension. My first reaction was to share her horror, judging the image against my naturalistic sense of where the uterus should be, that is, in its physiologic place. However, I began to realize that this organ was a psychological and symbolic one, and where it belonged was more a matter of the phenomenology of the soul-body than of the naturalistic one.

As we went on to explore this image, several complex new feelings and ideas emerged into awareness. Her first realization was that the uterus was that organ by which she could have children. The fact of it falling out led her to see directly what was horrifying to her; that in separating from her boyfriend, what would be lost was her opportunity to have a child. At this moment the wrenching deep within became acute, and this ache concretized her sense that without him, she would be barren and empty, for in him she vested her opportunity to give birth. She felt that in returning to school she might not meet anyone new and that would be the end of her hope for a child. Unconsciously she was being drawn down close to her belly, which helped her to look at her conflict: both wanting to be free and to stand alone, but not wanting to lose her opportunity for motherhood. Having literally made the decision to leave she felt her maternal possibility slipping away and in her panic and horror was grasping at it.

Further discussion led as well to the idea that it was not only the loss of the literal child that was horrifying but that, without her boyfriend, she could not be productive at all. Though she had set off for school and a new life, she felt her creative potential was dependent on him. Her relationship to her animus and therefore to important dimensions of her feminity remained unconscious.

It has been one of Jung's major contributions to the understanding of dreams to recognize that images not only point back to the past and reflect the present, but point to future possibilities as well. While the above images exposed her horror and fear of standing alone, it showed her that for the first time she held her feminity in her *own* hands! That is, the pathologized image's odd way of working in the soul conveyed an ironic sense of the soul's potentiality. It became a perspective through which she could view the events of her life, and gave her again a feeling for her possible agency and her potential to participate in her fate. The older depressive image of the feminine defined by her reproductive, rather than productive, potentials was falling away and was in a process of transformation. The sense that it was still possible to have children and be productive in other ways was there for her, and need not be embedded completely in an external man or left to the unconscious organ of her femininity lodged within her body. She had her hands on the numinous possibility of being a woman and on the organ of creation.

Erwin Straus (1966) has stated that when the hands are no longer asked to support and carry the body, they are relieved from their former duties and are free for new tasks. Here, psyche's hands hold the image of the feminine apart from its naturalistic and historical place, truly a condition of modern woman.

For thousands of years the place of the uterus, a woman's productive potential, was relegated to be within her body and within the unconscious. If it wandered, it was seen as a disease. Horowitz (1977) has documented how the notion of the displaced uterus belonged to the earliest recorded medicine in Egypt and Mesopotamia. The oldest medical text, the Kahun Papyrus, dates back to 1900 BC and describes the morbid states attributed to the displacement of the uterus. The physicians' efforts therefore, logically were directed toward returning it to its place from which it had strayed. Attempts were made to "drive down the uterus," and some of the methods used had the meaning of employing the image of a powerful male deity to lure back a wandering female organ. Horowitz, seeing the symbolic quality of this enactment, connects the "illness" to hysteria. But what is even more important is that we begin to develop new perspectives to see not only from a naturalistic viewpoint but from an imagistic one as well. The organs we speak of have psychic reality and in seeing them as such we cut ourselves free to recognize a more interior view of the soul's life.

Perhaps then it could be the case that physicians of soul might support a woman's desire that the powerful masculine within her cut free that organ of creation that may lead to childbearing and/or to the full range of human productivity. In any case, a modern woman would seem to have that possibility in her own grasp. For those of us who have come to see in dreams both an expression of the life of the soul and a narrative of its movements of the myriad complexities of affective and imagistic life, we must become aware that we are on a threshold not only of the new possibilities of the feminine, but of the larger possibilities of soul.

REFERENCES

Carrington, H., & Muldoon, S. (1929). *The projection of the astral body.* London: Rider & Co.

Hillman, J. (1975). *Re-visioning psychology.* New York: Harper & Row.

Horowitz, M. (Ed.). (1977). *Hysterical personality.* New York: Jason Aronson.

Straus, E. (1966). *Phenomenological psychology.* New York: Basic Books.

J. Greg Mogenson

Stepping Out of the Great Code

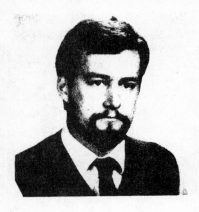

J. Greg Mogenseon is a marriage and family therapist practicing in the cities of Toronto and Stratford in Ontario. The present article is part of a book-length work now nearing completion titled "God is a Trauma: Psychoanalysis and Vicarious Religion."

220 Cobourg Street
Stratford, Ontario, Canada

I

After her suicide attempt, shortly before her release from the psychiatric hospital, she dreamed that she sat in a bathtub with light shining out of her nostrils. She found that she was able to take the batteries out of her head, disconnecting the light. The scene changed. Back in her apartment, sitting at a typewriter, she watched workers replace the glass window panes with white writing paper.

She told her friend the dream. He thought the dream psychotic. He thought that her ability to say the right things to the doctors to gain discharge from the hospital reflected less her sanity than her deftness at taking batteries out of her flashlight head. He told her that he believed the dream was suggesting that writing could provide a container for what her life could not contain.

Later that evening while reading Northrop Frye's (1981) book, *The Great Code: The Bible and Literature,* he came upon a passage that brought the dream she had told him back to mind. Writing about Leviathan, the great chaos monster of the oceans, Frye quotes a description of the creature from Job 41:18, "by his sneezings a light doth shine, and his eyelids are like the eyelids of the morning." Setting down the book, he pondered the connection between Leviathan and his friend's dream. "She is Leviathan," he thought. "Her psychosis is her identification with him. But how? How is it that this modern woman in a bathtub with batteries in her head manifests the chaos monster?"

He retired to bed, still preoccupied with this question. While sleeping, he dreamed. He was on the front lawn of his parents' home. Before him on the grass lay a bathtub. The bathtub was completely covered with crosses, Christian crosses. The crosses were drawn on the bathtub so densely that they formed together a cross-hatch or grid design. "Like

151

graph paper," he thought. Then he had a telephone in his hand. A man from England was on the line. The man said, "The anti-incarnational ideas you are now conceiving are very, very evil." The scene changed, amplifying the dream in other images. He was working on a fishing trawler. Huge catches of fish (fish = Christ) were being heaved on board in nets. The mesh of the nets reminded him of the crosses (or was this but an afterthought upon waking and recalling the dream?). Looking down at his legs he was fascinated to notice that his blue-jeans were entirely patterned with a graphic design of densely arranged crosses. Again the scene changed. He watched an artist make a grid of lines on a drawing. The grid of lines broke the picture into small units. The artist could then transpose the drawing to a larger grid or a smaller one, scaling the picture up or scaling it down.

In the morning he awoke full of dreams: hers from the day before and his own from the night past. "Jesus, the Incarnation," he thought, "it is through you that the spirit enters flesh, that Leviathan enters bathtubs and persons. Your cross scales the nonhuman, archetypal world down into man. Are you the carrier and source of the contagion from which we suffer?"

II

Wherever there is a gap in the human sphere a window festers open in the soul. An absent parent, a birth defect, the deficiencies of a modern education: we each have access to the stars through the avenue of our personal affliction. The child without a mother experiences the Great Mother in a less mediated fashion. He or she is no longer insulated from the archetype by its human carrier in his life. The individual with a physical deficit or organ inferiority, to use Adler's term, also tends to a more direct experience of the archetypes, creating consciousness in the precise shape of what is physically lacking and therefore psychically numinous. Likewise, the poorly educated experience the ubiquitous aspects of culture as unknown, numinous, disturbing, and fresh. These two worlds of experience shadow one another. The artifactual world, the world humans make (in relationships, in art, in science) rationalizes and attenuates the expression and experience of the other realm of being, the trans-human, archetypal world. Therapy mostly works with the artifactual. It aims at filling in the gaps in the human sphere, bringing families closer together or further apart, improving marital communication, increasing self-esteem. Were therapy, however, to address the realm of ideas and forms, conceiving of itself as a therapy of the archetype, culture would be moved in such a way that the human world would no longer require therapeutic maintenance because the cultural conditions that occasion its plight would be directly treated. The balm of intelligence, the dialogues spoken within the academy of the unhealed wound, would heal us by returning the culture

152

dumped upon us by the cultural collapse at aeons' end to its sources in the archetypes.

III

What happens when the culture is dumped upon the individual, when it no longer has the power to carry men and women, but is carried by them? William Blake praised the Bible, calling it "the Great Code of Art." Today, however, we recognize the Bible to be also the great code of psychopathology. Its stories have become thorns in our flesh. Its model has taken possession of the soul. If, as Jung (1960) said, "The gods have become diseases; Zeus no longer rules Olympus, but rather, the solar plexus" (par. 649), it is because the Christian model of God-incarnating has located him there. Today it is as if the only angels operative are fallen angels. No longer are there superordinate names, named categories of resemblances beyond the personal, to return to for perspective, context, and depth. Rahab, Behemoth, Leviathan; Judas, Lucifer, Jesus; Cain and Abel; Egypt and Jerusalem. Like the gold standard fluctuating behind the depressed dollar in our modern economic situation, these sacred standards, these digits of the Great Code, no longer back the substance of our lives in a healthy manner. Neurosis has appeared in the last century as a new covenant. Nauseous and empty, we are sickened with the psychic fallout of the Judeo-Christian promise torn loose from its supernatural moorings.

IV

The psyche or soul is an intermediary reality. In our Western (Neoplatonist) tradition it is the place "between" matter and spirit. Rarer than the physical world and more embodied than the spiritual world of purely intellectual forms, it is an imaginal world of metaphorical forms that image *how* the realms adjacent to it, matter and spirit commingle with one another.

In alchemy the soul was frequently spoken of as a mucilage or glue, and, indeed, all our soul-states express in imagination the ways in which the sacred and the profane are stuck together. Every fantasy, image, reflection, and metaphor, whether fluid in our minds and perception, or fixed into literature and art, colors our consciousness with descriptions of the relationship between the empirical world of our actual experience, and the spiritual world of our love, inspiration, and striving.

The political cartoon, for instance, articulates an intermediary reality, a pictorial of the soul. The doodle in the newspaper expresses in parody the gulf that holds the administrating spirit and the body politic together. Just a few squiggles of the cartoonist's pen and the presidents of the United States and the Soviet Union appear in their intermediate reality, playing soccer with the world. The biblical theme of Armageddon is relocated in contemporary events. World-destroying power rests in the hands of two mortals. In the excruciating exactness of a black-humored cartoon we witness a particular commingling of the sacred and the profane.

The intermediary reality of the soul can simply be sensed everywhere. The music of a friend's voice tells us how the message is to be taken. His or her inflections tell us what material and spiritual realities the words are struggling with. The whining, bitching, nasal tone; falsetto trembling; and body movements express one's personal connection to the otherwise objective meaning of one's sentences.

Peculiarities of style betray the shapes of our souls. The histrionics of the orator and the rhetoric of the writer are the persuasive stickinesses of the glue that binds the divine opposites together. Images have life and stimulate diverse responses, bringing the polarities into relationship in the eye of the beholder.

Of course, it may be objected that this so-called intermediary reality, or fictional level of existence, being at least in part an invented reality, does not lend itself to the kind of certainty that makes for valid science. Are the images we see and by which we see not essentially arbitrary? Is soul epistemology or ontology? Is it a hermeneutic method or a subtle kind of extended body? It is a map or a territory?

Questions such as these arise out of our philosophical responsibility to be objective. We want to be sure that we are not just seeing what we want to see. We want to know that our premises are weeded out of our conclusions, that our results are not invented, fudged. While these demands for objectivity may be the validity standards for other disciplines and other sciences, they can tend to obscure from psychology its empirical object, which is to say, itself. The scientific method is designed to keep the conventions and predispositions of our minds from influencing what is the object of investigation, out there before us in the test-tube. But, for psychology, the forms of the mind, its conventions and predilections, are the subject matter under investigation and when psychology employs the techniques of natural science it becomes, as Jung (1929/1967, par. 54) suggested, academic psychology, a psychology without the psyche. The science of soul—psychology—is a study of the biases, or determinate forms of subjectivity, both in the individual and in a collective, archetypal levels where we are all similar. The domain of psychology—its field of concern, its territory—is its maps. It is both epistemological—a method, a strategy of explication, and ontological—a realm of being, a place. The psyche is invented by individuals and inhabited by cultures. We invent our little bit of soul, but we come late in a long history of other makers. The psyche is both personal and collective, and the sources of our personal fictions are rooted in collective ones, cultural facts. No man is an island.

154

V

Feeling deeply betrayed by her husband's regression to his unlived adolescence soon after their marriage, she dreamed that she was in a barren desert with her husband and her father. The two men were naked. On one side of the van in which they had driven to the desert, her husband loaded beef carcasses into the vehicle; while on the other side, her father squatted as if to defecate, but instead of the expected bowel movement his genitals fell off. Passively, the dream-ego looked on as if she had nothing to do with the whole transaction.

Marriage, betrayal, husband, father, animal carcasses, castration—absent in their presence and present in their absence: How do they construct and deconstruct each other?

Marriage is a covenant, not only between a husband and a wife, but between the father of the bride and his son-in-law. In modern marriages the tradition still survives of the bride's father giving his daughter away. The two walk down the aisle together because the daughter is still considered the property of the father. But for the woman who dreamed this dream something had gone wrong with the marriage she had been given into, and she felt betrayed.

In biblical times promises were sworn over the testicles. When Abraham wanted his servant to take an oath he said to him, "put thy hand under my thigh" (Gen. 24:2). Castration images the breaking of a covenant. False testimonies break the promise of the testicles; covenants are broken in the groin.

The beef carcasses in the dream can also be referred to biblical notions of covenant. After a vision in which Yahweh proclaimed to Abraham his covenant with the Hebrew people assuring them a great future (Gen. 15:1), Abraham sacrificed an animal to him as an act of faith. That night in his dream Abraham saw "a smoking fire pot and a flaming torch" move between the pieces of the sacrificed animal. This dream of the ceremony of the covenant became a basic ritual in all contracts between people in ancient times. Covenants were sealed by sacrificing an animal and walking between the halves of its carcass. With this ritual the contractants demonstrated to one another that they would no more break their agreement than be cut in half like a sacrificed animal (Kelsey, 1974, p. 23).

In the dream the husband seizes the sacrifice while father looks on passively like a castrated shit. The feeling level of the dream seems to be saying: "Daddy, why didn't you save me from my husband? Why did you give me away without the promise and assurance of a good future? Father, you betrayed me by being taken in the bride-price deal; the imperfect covenant you made has caused me much, much pain."

On another level, however, these felt absences of the dream constellate presence. Her marriage is the sacrifice that takes her out of the father's genitals. By means of a series of separations and then finally a divorce, she broke out of the testicular prison of her patriarchal legacy. Buying herself a diamond ring, she handed herself over into her own hands. Now, paradoxically, marriage as an individual relationship—even to the same man—is possible. The personal friendship she maintains with her ex-husband is the new ground of a new culture. When the veil of marriage comes off the woman's face, the testicles come off the old father, and the two fundamental taboos of totemism (Freud 1913/1961) are left behind: the prohibition against individual relationships between men and women and the prohibition against breaking out of the superego structures of an extinct culture.

VI

We sometimes feel that our existence is insured, that the world owes us a living, that nothing untoward could happen to us. At other times we may feel, to the contrary, that we are cosmic orphans, disinherited by the world's malevolent god. The archetype of the covenant, the promise between God and his people—between the Self and ourselves—can constellate both positively and negatively in our lives. We feel the polarity of the archetype: security/insecurity, trust/mistrust, positive father/negative father.

When therapy is influenced by the conventional theological thinking surrounding this archetype it tends to adopt theology's goal of reconciliation. The negative father-complex must be made positive by reframing the superego through love and the Israel of its promise. By hook or crook, halfway house, Big Brothers, or Tough Love, the prodigal son must go home and meet the father.

So many therapy hours are devoted to untangling and reforming human communication, the words and phrases that composed the lived covenants in which love is supposed to be shared. Transactional Analysis, in particular, has tried to convert its clients to this Zionism called "contractual living." The *Word* becomes flesh and a humanistic communion is celebrated in the sharing of relationship-bound feelings in a therapy group. However, when the goal of therapy is realizing archetypes and differentiating among them, the incarnational model of therapy can be seen to imply a loss of psychological acuity (the incarnation of the one requiring the sacrifice of the many). We can no longer perceive the archetypal dimension of our engagements when we seek psyche only in contractual relationships governed by covenantal assertions: I'm O.K./you're O.K.; he's a distractor, she's an avoider; Jungians are mystifiers.

From the archetypal perspective, the language of covenant, oath, and law represses the anima even as Brunnhilde is imprisoned in Woton's ring of fire and Aphrodite-Venus in Uranus's genitalia. There is a fundamental contradiction between living a psychic life where anima is turned toward the archetypes and living a humanistic life where anima is confined within a logos of agreements. In this latter situation the anima is imprisoned in our physical, incarnational, communal life. The psyche is literalized. However, when we approach the psyche non-incarnationally (Gnostically) and the anima is free to relate us to the stars, it does not mean the human level is ignored. Rather, it means that the human is restored to a relative position among the other archetypes. Our exaggerated preoccupation with human relationships—not lack of human science—creates the afflictions we suffer within our human world.

VII

He went to a lecture at the University on the poetry of the English Romantics. The lecturer suggested that the theme of Romanticism, whatever its content, was the process of its own making. The poets, he said, were writing about writing. They were trying to build a temple for the soul "Where branched thoughts, new grown with pleasant pain,/Instead of pines shall murmur in the wind." The lecturer quoted from John Keats' (1958) famous letter:

> Call the world if you Please "The vale of Soul-making." Then you will find out the use of the world (I am speaking now in the highest terms for human nature admitting it to be immortal which I will here take for granted for the purpose of showing a thought which has. struck me concerning it). I say *"Soul-making"* Soul as distinguished from an Intelligence—There may be intelligences or sparks of divinity in millions—but they are not Souls till they acquire identities, till each one is personally itself. I[n]telligences are atoms of perception—they know and they see and they are pure, in short they are God—How then are Souls to be made? How then are these sparks which are God to have identity given them—so as ever to possess a bliss peculiar to each one's individual existence? How, but by the medium of a world like this? This point I sincerely wish to consider because I think it a grander system of salvation than the Chrystean religion. (p. 288)

Later that night, at home in bed, he drifted off into the culture, he drifted off into a dream. On the lawn beside St. Paul's Anglican Church a tent was pitched and tightly zippered up. In the grass around the tent lay money—loose coins, change. He was with friends. He and they were local boys. They were maverick, delinquent, and uproarious. The scene changed. He was listening to a repetition of last evening's lecture on the Romantic poets. While the lecturer spoke he held the dreamer's head tightly between his hands. This show of affection was slightly embarrassing to the dreamer. At last, the lecturer released his hold and the dreamer swooned. The hands had been holding the dreamer's head very tightly, cutting off the blood. The dreamer struggled to remain conscious and did manage to keep his wits. Then he noticed an article written by the lecturer titled, "Elegy." With the article was a polemic by a literary critic condemning the piece as mad or evil. Female custodians, fascinated with the lecture, allowed the talk to go on past the University's closing time. Finally, the lecture ended and the lecturer invited a dark woman to join him and they left together. Then the time orientation shifted back to the middle of the lecture. The dreamer left the lecture hall, perhaps to use a washroom, perhaps because he was still dizzy from the lecturer's hold on his head. He entered a very small room or cell. The walls were old and covered with graffiti. A single, naked, light-bulb hung down as a source of light. Reaching down into his trousers he examined his scrotum. He felt his testicles and found with them in his scrotum a third one and a fourth. Then a voice said flatly and with objective intonation: "The god of the Christian religion is no god at all." Over and over again the voice repeated the statement: "The god of the Christian religion is no god at all." He thought it important to remember the statement. Beside him on the floor there was some cheap, newsprint-quality paper. With a pen he started to write down the sentence—"The god of the Christian religion"— but before he could write the whole sentence down the earliest words began to vanish. The paper wouldn't take the ink. Again he tried to write the sentence down. Again and again. But the ink would not take. He noticed, however, that as he wrote the paper became of finer and finer quality until at last it attained a satin finish. Worried that he was going mad and that he would not be able to find his way out of the little closet (or even record the sentence that might hold the key to releasing him) he awoke with a fright.

After hearing a lecture on the Romantics, after hearing how Wordsworth tapped the hiding places of power for the refreshment of his soul's life, the dreamer finds himself in the yard outside St. Paul's Anglican Church even as Coleridge, in his Mariner's Rime, let himself slip "below the Kirk, below the hill, below the lighthouse top" to the well-springs of the creative imagination. When the dreamer resides outside the Church among his Gnostic brethren in the vale of Soul-making there is money in the grass, loose change. In the vale of Soul-making, in that place of a salvation grander than that of the "Chrysteain religion," change is loosed and value freed from the sacramental containers of the Church.

Inside the lecture hall the contents of the dreamer's head push out even as the lecturer's hands squeeze in around it and tighten the focus. The pressure in the dreamer's head builds up like the multiplication of the loose change in the grass and makes him dizzy. He swoons and nearly passes out. The Romantic vision of the possibilities of Soul-making is releasing his soul from its Christian parameters. An article titled "Elegy" catches the dreamer's attention. The lecturer is reciting an elegy. He is releasing the imagination by announcing the death of its old containers: the Christian Church and the Christian god.

The soul's release is the feminine's return. The female custodians step out of their janitorial roles, enter the Academy, and listen to the talk. Their release from patriarchal domination is what Soul-making is all about. A fundamental taboo of totemism has been removed. The lecturer and the dark woman go off together as equals.

In the middle of the whole process the dreamer leaves the lecture hall and, in a small cell or closet covered with the genital grammar (graffiti) of patriarchy, takes down his trousers and examines his testicles. There are four of them. Abraham and servant (Gen. 24:2), the whole covenantal tradition of the divine word and promise, is emerging in his scrotum. Money in the grass, pressure in the head, a doubling of the testicles: Each image is a commentary on the others. No longer are there testicles above him. The testicles of God, like the tablets of Moses, have smashed to pieces like loose change in the grass. The soul has been released from the reified, codified, authorized traditions of the spirit into the multiple and individual possibilities of the imagination and making. Like Aphrodite-Venus emerging from the severed testicles of the sky-father Uranus, the female custodians and the dark woman emerge also. Charwomen are now sages.

"The god of the Christian religion is no god at all." The sentence is a declaration of freedom, freedom from the genital grammar of monotheistic tyranny. Any god who takes the imagination captive is no god at all.

He tries to write the sentence down but he cannot. The ink will not take. Again he tries and again. He worries that he is going mad. Without god, without boundaries and limiting structures, there is uncertainty. Anything is possible. Perhaps, he thinks, simply writing down the declaration that the god is no god will give him a point of certainty, a standpoint. But Soul-making will not be reified into truth-statements. The new wine will not be placed in the old bottles. With every sentence that will not take to the page the dreamer is further abandoned to the process of writing and to the uncertainties of the imagination (the question: What does the soul want?). Again and again he tries to write down a positive declaration and each time the sentence vanishes. Over time, however, the paper transforms, becoming of better and better quality. The dreamer's soul, by long apprenticeship to uncertainty, coagulates into the substantiality and quality of satin-finish paper. It is precisely this process of interminable writing or Soul-making that is the dreamer's way of stepping over the patriarchal threshold and out of the Great Code.

VIIII

"No one comes to the Father but by the Son." With this statement the oracles were stilled (John Milton). No longer could Delphi give us diagnosis. No longer could we find the altars specific to our afflictions and concerns. The *ta'wil,* the Return, the re-collection and re-cognition of archetypes, gods, and myths was absorbed into a single instance of it, the Christian one. Incarnation, crucifixion, resurrection, and apocalypse became the model for our experience and response to all events and happenings. After 2,000 years of Christian reductionism, a millenium of thoughts and thorns, tastes and experiences have been taken prisoner for Christ.

REFERENCES

Freud, S. (1961). Totem and taboo. In J. Strachey (Ed. and Trans.), *The standard edition of the complete psychological works of Sigmund Freud* (Vol. 13, pp. 1-161). London: Hogarth Press. (Original work published 1913).

Frye, N. (1981). *The great code: The bible and literature.* New York: Harcourt Brace.

Keats, J. (1958). *Selected poems and letters* (D. Bush, Ed.). Boston: Houghton Mifflin.

Jung, C. G. (1960). The structure and dynamics of the psyche. In H. Read, M. Fordham, & G. Adler (Eds.) and R. Hull (Trans.), *The collected works of C. G. Jung* (Vol. 8). Princeton: Princeton University Press/Bollingen Series XX. (Original work published 1931).

Jung, C. G. (1967). Alchemical studies. In H. Read, M. Fordham, & G. Adler (Eds.) and R. Hull (Trans.) *The collected work of C. G. Jung* (Vol. 13). Princeton: Princeton University Press/Bollingen Series XX. (Original work published 1929).

Kelsey, M. T. (1974). *God, dreams, and revelation.* Minneapolis: Augsburg Publishing House.

Luis Raul Rios-Garcia

The Pelican and the Flamingo:

A Therapist's Dreams in the Process of Self-Exploration

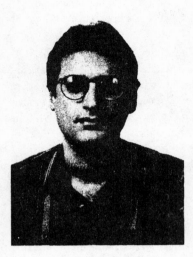

I was born in Puerto Rico, lived in Spain during my childhood, and completed graduate degrees in clinical psychology in the United States. Now back in Puerto Rico, I am mostly involved in family therapy as a clinician and teacher, within a general hospital and in a small private practice. Most of my free time is spent joyously with my wife, Maria, 8-year-old Alejandra, and 7-year-old Gabriel. Another recent source of enjoyment and fun is my involvement as a pianist with a jazz quintet.

Centro de Desarrollo Personal
El Monte Mall—Suite 23—Tercer Piso
Avenida Muños Rivera
Hato Rey, Puerto Rico 00918

The connection between personal and professional growth was not clear to me, or understood by me, until very recently. In previous years, the development of my professional skills took priority, rather artificially, over my personal growth, with subsequent unbalanced results. This process of disharmony, in addition to recent stress precipitated by a physical relocation, led to my rediscovery of dreams as a tool for self-exploration. My dreams have simultaneously illustrated a growth process through images and metaphors and provided the sense of personal direction and meaning needed to reestablish balance in a creative way. As we therapists foster self-discovery in ourselves through disciplined examination of our own lives and dreams, we communicate an attitude favorable to self-exploration in our patients.

Dreams have been described classically as the royal road to the unconscious, but also as the soil from which most symbols originally grow (Jung, 1964), and as the primary intuitive mode of consciousness (Ornstein, 1977). What is mysterious and attractive about dreams is their apparently illogical, incoherent, metaphorical, and rich imagery. My own approach to dreams is existential and Jungian. In addition, I apply my studies of oriental philosophy to the understanding of dreams and the process of change.

From existentialists I have learned that dreams are intrinsically meaningful experiences of being-in-the-world, equally real and valid as waking experiences. Secondly, existence is revealed through contingency, absurdity, and anxiety—three common themes of dreams. Thus, dreams mirror the existential situation or circumstances of the moment.

Jungian writers state that dreams reveal the basic connections between our personal unconscious and the archetypal images of the collective unconscious, by way of the language of symbolism. They also provide cues to the proper balance of inner and outer psychic experience and point toward resolution of conflict.

Finally, the *I Ching* or Book of Changes (Wilhelm, 1967), an ancient treatise of practical wisdom, can be used as a method for exploring the unconscious. Its 64 hexagrams are quite rich in content, suggesting a wealth of symbols and images that relate to everyday situations. My use of the *I Ching* in this paper assumes the principle of synchronicity which, according to Jung, "takes the coincidence of events in space and time as meaning something more than mere chance" (Foreword to the *I Ching*). In addition to philosophical wisdom, the hexagrams in the *I Ching*, through their images and symbols, amplify those images present in my dreams.

The dreams that follow are a sample of six dreams from a total of 125 that were recorded during a period of 2 years. During this time my family and I relocated from the island of Puerto Rico, our Motherland, to the city of Los Angeles. These dreams focus specifically on the experience and the process of growth precipitated by this relocation: the journey of the soul and the search for centeredness and inner balance. The images and metaphors revealed in these dreams have been present at other times in my life, but never with such intensity and consistency. The six dreams speak for themselves, but their manifest content will sometimes suggest specific associations and background information, which will be presented accordingly, as commentaries. Therefore, rather than follow the traditional clinical style where background data are usually presented first, the dreams themselves will lead the way. They are presented thematically, not chronologically.

The Dreams

This first dream illustrates the issue of competence in relation to a new unfamiliar task in a new setting.

Dream 1: The Hawk: This is a squad of Los Angeles policeman (a group of four or five). I am *The Hawk,* the leader. The squad gets on a futuristic, electronic vehicle, much like a small subway car. However, rather than moving along tracks, this vehicle (or spaceship) moves through the air. We are surprised; we did not expect the vehicle to fly. I am the pilot. Like a car, it has two pedals, side by side; one for acceleration on the right, and the break on the left. At first I have great difficulty with the controls. I can't seem to get it right. When I try to depress the acceleration pedal so that the vehicle soars through the air, my foot gets entangled under the pedal. It takes a while to coordinate this movement.

162

Finally, I manage to step on it, and the vehicle shoots up. We fly by the Los Angeles downtown skyline, at night, gracefully, between the buildings. I feel satisfied. Our task is to fly over the coliseum, or sports arena, in order to position ourselves in front of a big, newly constructed condominium building. The building is a luxurious apartment complex with marble walls, huge columns, and beautiful plants hanging from the balconies. We are headed in that direction. Again I start to maneuver the pedals, with some confusion, but quickly get control of the vehicle. Slowly, we rise above the city until we find the building and position ourselves in front of it. I experience a great sense of satisfaction and accomplishment as I admire the building and fly around it.[1]

Commentary. Two years ago, I experienced the burnout syndrome in all its dimensions. For many months, my self-worth was defined almost exclusively by my work as a psychologist, to the extent of overwork, and with the subsequent denial. As a prelude to this process, following graduate school, I had attempted to become a model father, husband, and son, as well as an all-around clinician: private practice; professor; consultant to multiple programs; and specialist in difficult patient populations, such as terminal patients, substance abusers, and acute schizophrenics. The result was professional achievement coupled with personal exhaustion and alienation from others. The dream addresses the question of the need to find a new, balanced way of feeling competent as a person and as a professional in a new setting.

Of particular importance in the dream is the necessity to coordinate the left and right pedals in order for the work to be done. Thus, an issue in my own personal growth, as well as in my development as a therapist, has to do with the proper balance between two basic polarities: the intellectual, analytical, linear, forward mode of experience; and the intuitive, holistic, nonlinear, receptive mode. It is apparent that crude attempts to control my performance by awareness about external circumstances and compliance with them, in the absence of a true integration of these two experiencing modes, leads to obstruction and defeat. Thus, the more we seek to maintain ego control of our performance, the more anxious we become and the more our natural, intuitive skills are blocked.

A Deeper Search for the Hidden Soul: The Child as Guide

The following dreams reflect rebirth, change, and the turmoil associated with this: they foretell transformation at a deeper level.

---

1. The similarity between the imagery revealed in this dream and that of a recent motion picture, *Blade Runner*, is illustrative of the principle of synchronicity. Watching the movie three years after having experienced this dream enlightened the personal meaning of these images. I felt alien, and overwhelmed, but oddly competent.

Dream 2: A visit to the asylum. This is a nightmare—a very long, confusing, haunting vision. Though the first part is not clear, at the conclusion of the dream I am entering a building. A mysterious, enigmatic child is leading me inside. He reminds me of my son, Gabriel, but, unlike my son, he has black hair. He leads me down a long, narrow, somber hall. He knows where he is going, so I follow. The child says nothing, but occasionally he turns around to see if I am behind him and smiles mysteriously, diabolically. He just continues to walk slowly ahead. As we progress down the hall, I get more and more frightened. The halls resemble those of an asylum. Patients enter the hall, like ghosts; we pass very near their faces and I can see them, feel their presence. I sense they are coming toward me, grimacing, making horrible faces, laughing. But they do not touch me, they just pass me by. I am very frightened but, at the same time, I feel the child knows where he is going, so I trust him. I sense that the process of going is more frightening than the destination. It does not matter where we are going. . . .

Dream 3: Cherish and protect the orphan child. The setting is World War II. Death and destruction are all around. A nurse is rounding up a group of orphan children to take them to a refuge. They arrive. The refuge is a ravaged building in ruins. Only the foundations are intact. A Puerto Rican soldier is desperately looking for a bit of humanity amid so much destruction. The nurse takes the children down to a basement using an improvised elevator; she wants to hide them. The soldier befriends one of the orphans, an 8-year-old boy. He names the child Harlequin. The soldier wants to protect him from war; he hides him in the basement, among the ruins, "Stay quiet, don't move, the enemy might be coming." Although the basement is in ruins, light is coming through the windows. The soldier searches for his rifle; he has bullets but he can't find his rifle. He does not want to fight anymore. He senses the tension building up. He wants to be safe, and wants the child to be safe, but knows they are no longer secure in the basement. He searches for the orphan in order to flee: "Harlequin! Harlequin!" There is no answer until, finally, the child comes out of the ruins. "Come on, let's go, hurry." At this moment, they see a band of mercenaries who come to loot and murder. But the soldier doesn't have a rifle: he doesn't know how to protect the orphan. They will have to hide among the ruins and hope that they are not discovered. But he fears they have already been spotted. Maybe he will have to fight. He wants to protect the child, but he doesn't know how. He is frightened.

Dream 4: The earthquake. My mother, my daughter, Alejandra, and I are living in a one-bedroom apartment in Los Angeles. It is made of wood and plaster, like most dwellings here. Mother has gone out and Alejandra is playing in the front yard, dressed in a nice, long summer dress. I am inside. Walking toward the back of the building, I see my

164

mother coming toward me, carrying grocery bags. Suddenly, there is a severe earthsquake. This is the big one. As I look, in shock, I see movement in the walls around me. Everything is turning around with great force and speed, like a very fast merry-go-round. I am paralyzed. After a few minutes, I run toward the front door to see if my daughter is all right. At this time, the whole apartment is pushed forward violently as if shaven off its base, and tumbles right into an immense crack on the ground in the front yard. There is destruction all around us. Before falling into the open ground, I look up and see the Los Angeles City Hall building crumble. I feel myself falling into the crack, with my daughter. Miraculously, nothing has happened to us; we are not hurt. We come out of the ground, and when I look at Alejandra, she has turned black.

Commentary. In discussing the eight basic triagrams of the *I Ching,* and Taoist philosophy, Wilhem and Jung (1962) tell us that the marriage of *K'an* (the water, the abysmal, eros) and *Li* (sun, fire, logos) produces the child, the new person. Jungians, reflecting the wisdom of ancient mythology, regard the child as a symbol of rebirth, the creative spirit which provides the energy for the release from conventional, rational ways of being to new, progressive ones. It is a symbol of both the regressive and the progressive direction in discovery. In the first two dreams (dreams 2 and 3) we see the duality in symbolism: First, we encounter the child as providing guidance, leading me into the frightening, deep recesses of my psyche. I am a passive follower. In the second dream I am actively meeting my child and actively attempting to guard him, to protect him from outer reality, which is fearful and disturbing. The last dream, the image of the earthquake, shakes my very being, my psychic house, and sends me deep into my soul. Thus, the message is that transformation is not possible without crisis, tension, and agitation of the very foundations of our being.

Beginning of an Integration

Release from bondage, and exploration of new ways of being are the central themes of this final section.

Dream 5: The strange animal in the park. My family and I are riding in the back of a truck, on a tour. We are being shown the animals in the zoo. We are driving on a dirt road with green wooded areas at both sides. The children are really excited, and so am I. We have seen a few animals already. Now, we come to the grizzly bears. We see them at the right side of the road and stop. They are black, and they look ferocious. As we approach them, they growl, revealing their deadly fangs. The children calmly pick up some grass and feed the bears, naturally, with no apparent fear. I am surprised, but I follow them and do the same thing.

165

Back on the truck we continue down the road. Then we see the rest of the bears, sleeping soundly on the grass under the shadow of the trees. We continue the tour. I am expecting something unknown. I have the feeling this is just the beginning; we are going to see the *real* animal soon. Several minutes pass, and suddenly, a strange animal comes hopping out of the woods and crosses our path. We have to maneuver the truck to avoid hitting him. We come up to him—he is at our left side and we get a good look at him. He is a cross between a moose, a kangaroo, and a man. His body is that of a strong, muscular man, totally white, as if bathed in milk. He has a moose's head and his legs and long tail clearly resemble those of a kangaroo. He is hopping, with his two legs joined together, like a kangaroo, in a very graceful, precise way. As we get near him, he greets us with a loud, inhuman, painful scream, and he disappears into the forest. We respond with amazement, and then continue on our way. I am very impressed by this creature. Although he is suffering, I presume, because of his inability to walk, he jumps the best way he can, gracefully and self-assured. He makes the best of it.

Dream 6: The pelican and the flamingo. Sitting on the rocks by the seashore on a gray winter day, we are interviewing what seems to be a pelican, although his wings are short and his legs are long and thin, like a flamingo's. Actually, he is a cross between these two birds. The animal tells us about his misfortune. He is a tropical creature, but he is living here now. He tells us about his weakness in that his legs are fragile, likely to bend easily. It is difficult for him to feed himself, to procure his own nourishment. Although he eats marine organisms, he depends on humans for feeding. He is a large, awkward bird, like a flamingo. Thus, he doesn't have the pelican's agility in that he cannot just dive for fish; his long legs get in the way. I visualize the bird in a man-made pool, eating what people feed him. I ask, "Can't you fly, and emigrate." "No, my wings are too short; we don't emigrate. We wait for the arrival of the summer, when it is hot and things improve. Then we can fly and search for our own food." I think to myself, "He's going to wait for the summer to arrive, wait for his time." Then, I have the image of him flying effortlessly, gracefully.

Commentary. Specific associations to these two dreams are as follows. The strange creature's scream reminds me of an experience I had during Zen meditation 6 years ago. During the third sitting on a given evening of group meditation, I was startled by a very loud scream. Later on, questioning the other participants I learned that nobody else had heard it. The experience was so frightening that I could not meditate again for many months and, even then, not to the extent or depth of that time. I have understood since then that the scream came from deep within my soul and, like the creature in the dream, signaled perhaps the need for release from bondage of a primitive, instinctual, potent side of me—my "left" side, which has long been denied. The man-moose-kangaroo is a metaphor revealing the need to give this side a voice, in order to reclaim its proper place in my total psyche. In this manner, it points toward initial attempts at an integration.

Secondly, the pelican reminds me of those beautiful animals of the sea that I have seen and photographed during summer sailing trips in the Caribbean waters. I have always been impressed by their agility, the precision with which they dive for their prey. Likewise, I associate the flamingo with softness, grace, and calm, together with awkwardness in flying. At another level, the embodiment of the pelican and the flamingo in a single creature is for me a metaphor of the therapist. As therapists, we combine grace and softness in intention and manner with accuracy and precision in technique. Summer, furthermore, is full of bloom and signifies rebirth; being from the Caribbean, it is the *natural* season for me. Although first in bondage and dependent, the bird releases itself by keeping in touch with nature. This, then, is the message for further growth.

Postscript: The Process of Growth Revisited

The preceding dreams reveal a variety of images, metaphors, and symbols that, in terms of content, suggest common themes in my personal and professional life. They manifest the search for the soul as an inner journey synchronous with the outer journey from one country to another. But they also point to a process characteristic of all human beings in transition toward expansion of awareness, and growth. Rossi (1972) has outlined a series of stages in this process. He asserts that dreams reveal the path through these stages and, therefore, are good indicators to progress. As a way of concluding, I will attempt to illustrate how some of these dreams (or parts of them) correspond to these stages.

In the initial stages, according to Rossi, the dreamer experiences himself or herself as thrust into a new unpredictable situation, and then begins to feel blocked. There is a lack of awareness of our own uniqueness and a frightening attitude toward the new. A sense of confusion, loss of control, and inadequacy are revealed. My experience of being guided by the mysterious child in *A visit to the asylum* and the initial parts of *The hawk* are illustrative of this experience. Further into the process, we encounter crisis, which reflects conflict between the emerging awareness and the older world view. The old, unidimensional existence is shattered. Dreams typically reflect war, danger, and destruction *thema*. *Cherish and protect the orphan child* and *The earthquake* are examples of this stage. The final stages of growth concern the synthesis of new awareness and reality. First, we acknowledge the autonomous transformation that is taking place; multiple levels of awareness coexist with one another. Then, we learn to use the newfound awareness. In Rossi's own words, "The natural process of growth and transformation are integrated with our conscious, self-directed efforts to change in a particular direction" (p. 19). *The hawk* represents the best illustration, perhaps, of all these stages. After an initial period of confusion and disorganization, I become aware of the way to direct the space vehicle to the goal, experiment with it, and finally achieve it. Likewise, the pelican-flamingo is waiting for his time to actualize his flight and autonomy, and the man-moose-kangaroo is a metaphor for such a synthesis. The final stages also concern themselves with a creative relationship to ourselves and others. Here we can easily translate our new awareness into *actual,* more creative ways of being, experiencing, feeling, behaving differently. The soul is rediscovered, and this gives a transcendental dimension to the process of growth. As new challenges are met, the growth cycle summarized in these stages repeats itself, and one is never the same after each of these cycles.

Many of the personal issues stirred up in this paper are still relevant. The struggle is still going on. The process must unfold, take its natural course, in the direction that these dreams provide. Our challenge as therapists is to create an optimal balance between inner and outer reality, expressed in a synthesis of our personal and professional lives.

REFERENCES

Harding, M. E. (1973). *The I and the not-I: A study in the development of consciousness.* Princeton: Princeton University Press (Bollingen Series).

Jung, C. G. (1964). Approaching the unconscious. In C. G. Jung (Ed.), *Man and his symbols* (pp. 18-103). New York: Dell.

Ornstein, R. (1977). *The psychology of consciousness.* New York: Harcourt, Brace, Janovich.

Rossi, E. L. (1972). *Dreams and the growth of personality: Expanding awareness in psychotherapy.* New York: Pergamon Press.

van der Post, L. (1975). *Jung and the story of our time.* New York: Vintage Books.

Wilhelm, R. (1967). *The I Ching, or book of changes.* Princeton: Princeton University Press (Bollingen Series).

Wilhelm, R., & Jung, C. G. (1962). *The secret of the golden flower: A Chinese book of life.* New York: Harcourt, Brace, Janovich.

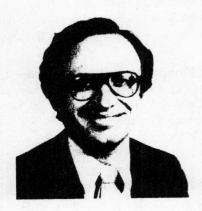

Meyer Rohtbart

A Vital Person in My Life and An Experience of Synchronicity

I am a psychiatrist in private practice interested in the interplay of humor, religion, and psychotherapy. I work as a hospital clown and teach clowns to work with hospitalized psychiatric patients. I also teach a pastoral counseling course for The Reconstructionist Rabbinal College.

My personal pleasures include being married, playing with my two children, community activities, and tennis.

One Bala Avenue
Bala Cynwyd, Pennsylvania 19004

Connie Young sounds like Carl Jung. The spelling is different, the sound the same.

Connie was my high-school English Literature teacher (Oak Park High School, Class of 1963) and she became very special to me. She responded to me when I was confused and hurt, having just broken up with a girl. My family would have disapproved of the relationship. I ended it before they could find out and before I could find out just how attached I had become.

I was in the library, distracted, when Connie asked personally and quietly, "Is something wrong? I'm interested." So I shared this story and other intimate stories about me. It was easy. She expressed her love by listening intently and responding emotionally. I had never spoken to anyone like her before and found it soothing. She said, "I think psychotherapy could help you." So I clandestinely went to therapy using Bar Mitzvah savings. She said, "I think you could be a wonderful psychiatrist—you are compassionate." So I volunteered to work for a child psychiatrist during summer vacation. She said, "I think you should go away to college, it will help you develop." So I did that too, and when my father died she gave me the name of a psychiatrist in New York who turned out to be her former therapist.

Then it was time for medical school. I felt enslaved. I wanted to quit. My family panicked. I panicked. Connie consoled me. She didn't much care what I did as long as I kept my integrity. I found my integrity and decided to finish my freshman year. Fortunately, this was the end of Connie's crisis intervention. I began to feel a shift in our relationship toward becoming more of a peer and we enjoyed each other. I'm glad I took care of the logistics of getting her to my wedding. Giving to her was becoming more important to me as she was now approaching 70 years of age. She was 75 years old when I finished my psychiatry residency. Whenever I visited her, we spent most of our time talking about psychology, religion, and our families. (She had never married.) These talks were affectionate, lively, and interesting.

Then, at age 80, 5 years ago, her health began to fail her. She was deeply religious and this, along with her several dear friends, sustained her. At one point, she had been demoralized for quite some time. She had lost some vision and reading was becoming a chore. She was not eating well. I was planning to see her in 2 months. I called to tell her that and she told me she didn't know if she would still be around. I felt inspired and made a dinner date for the following Saturday night and took her to her favorite restaurant. It helped her appetite and my ego.

I last saw Connie when my wife and I took her to my 20th-Year High School Reunion. She was vibrant. She was the only teacher there and she saw many former pupils. Her memories came alive.

Connie died Monday, June 24, 1985, at the age of 85. I found out as my wife, Judy, took me to the airport en route to the American Academy of Psychotherapists Summer Workshop. I was upset and denied it. After all, Connie and I had said good-bye a number of times and she had even given me some "inheritance" gifts. At the opening dinner, I sat with a number of people from my ongoing group. Also at the table, sitting next to me on my right was a therapist named Lucille, who lived in Oak Park, Michigan, of all places. She knew Connie and asked me if I knew that she had just died. We both were amazed at the "coincidence."

Synchronicity: an acausal connecting principle. It is all pretty subjective—or is it? I feel a sense of meaningful mystery in addition to sadness at my loss.

The mystery is in the ways that Connie's death intersected with AAP and *VOICES* as well as my writing process. I rarely write papers. The editorial deadline for articles related to Jung was extended at that AAP Workshop. Meeting Lucille at the opening AAP dinner, realizing that Jung sounded like Young, and knowing that my relationship to Connie developed values that led to AAP, impelled me to write. I often wrote for Connie as a high-school student and find myself wishing she could read this.

It's been difficult to end this paper. I feel confused. Why is it so painful for Connie to be gone? We said good-bye many times and appreciated each other very often explicitly in word and deed. Her life was a celebration and she is a welcome part of me. So why is it so difficult? My left brain knows and that may prove valuable in time.

Robert M. Stein

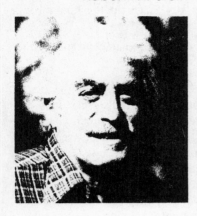

The Incest Wound and the Marriage Archetype*

Robert M. Stein, M.D., is a Jungian analyst in private practice in Los Angeles. He received his Diplomate in Analytical Psychology from the C. G. Jung Institute in Zurich in 1959. He is the author of many published papers, but is best known for his original psychological study of the incest mystery, *Incest and Human Love,* Spring Publications, 1984, which has also been published in many languages.

450 North Bedford Drive—Suite 303
Beverly Hills, California 90210

I

I shall begin with the notion that *human psychological development is dependent on the sense of incompletion and the desire for completion.* Plato (1952) expressed this same idea in mythic form: Originally the gods created man round and totally self contained; with four hands, four feet, and one head with two identical faces looking in opposite directions and set on a round neck. Some of these original men were given both male and female genitalia, while others received two sets of identical genitals, either all male or all female. They were enormously powerful and able to move with incredible speed by leaping into cart-wheel turns with their four hands and four feet. The gods were delighted with their creation until one day these round men became so inflated with their own strength and power that they made an attack upon the gods. Whereupon Zeus, realizing his mistake, cut them in half and ever since we have been searching for our missing other half.

Psychologically, this notion that each of us must find our soul-mate for completion is directly related to the mystery surrounding the taboo against incest. The incest taboo is universal. Kroeber (1959) and other anthropologists have suggested that it is the only universal human institution. We do not know the origins of the incest taboo. Freud and his followers view the taboo as entirely a product of culture. Following the archetypal perspective,[1] I have developed the view that *both the incest*

---

* This article originally appeared in the November 1984 issue of *HARVEST,* Journal of the Analytical Psychology Club, London. Editor, Joel Rye-Menuhin, M. Phil. (Lond.). Reprinted with permission.

1. The archetypal perspective presupposes that all the typical human modes of being and behavior as well as all the social forms and institutions of culture, are instinctually rooted even though they may eventually become oppressive to the evolution of the human spirit.

desire and the taboo are instinctually rooted, and that the tension between the desire and the inhibition functions as a key factor in the humanizing process of psychological development by:

1. stimulating us to an awareness of our incompleteness and to the desire for completion;

2. activating our sexual imagination. (Stein, 1984).

Both Freud and Jung see the inhibition of the child's incestuous desires to have intercourse with the parent as the primary function of the incest taboo. They view the desire between brother and sister as secondary extensions of the drive for union with the parent. In my book, *Incest and Human Love* (Stein, 1984), I have questioned this emphasis. The Polynesian verb *tapui,* from which the word *tabu* originates, means "to make holy," "to set apart." In this way an object is endowed with mana and numinosity. By sanctifying or deifying the parental relationship, the taboo creates a psychological distance which is essential for the development of consciousness. An aura of mystery begins to surround the parents, stimulating the child's imagination to focus on the special qualities of mother and father and their relationship. This unique human veneration of the parents stimulates the release of the archetypal image of the Sacred Marriage (*hieros gamos*) and of the child's first experience of its human incarnation. This image, which Jung (1955/1963) has called the Incest Archetype, expresses the harmonious union and polarity between the masculine-feminine opposite, a root metaphor for the union of all opposites. Jung describes this archetype as an image of the supreme union of opposites expressed as a combination of things which are related but of unlike nature.

When this image becomes obscured or lost, life loses all meaning and consequently its balance. Without an incest taboo toward the parents it is doubtful that culture would have developed, but I do not believe the taboo is essential for prevention of sexual union between parent and child—parental instincts, even among animals, are generally sufficient to prevent this. In the brother-sister relationship, however, the taboo is crucial in preventing sexual involvement. Primitive societies have developed elaborate and stringent rituals designed to prevent sexual contact between brother and sister. For example, they are not allowed to speak in any personal or intimate way after a certain age, or to look at each other in public, or even to sit on the same mat until they are very old. On the other hand, a deep love and respect for each other is cultivated within the family—in a patrilineal culture the brother is even responsible for the welfare of his sister and her children. This combination of a deep bond and the impossibility of personal involvement stimulates the child's interest and imagination in this fascinating, look-alike contemporary.

A boy will experience his sister as closely related to his being, yet she is an unknown "holy" other, forever unattainable. He is dedicated to loving and serving her, but he can never unite with her. The same experience applies to a girl in relation to her brother. The longing to find and to unite with the mysterious other half of oneself is a direct consequence of the brother-sister taboo. This uniquely human attribute is largely responsible for man's eternal fascination with all matters concerning love, sex, and the human connection. It has helped transform the sexual drive from a purely biological urge to the supreme instrument of man's psychological development. Above all, in his longing to find his soul-mate, man is able ultimately to discover and shape his own soul.

The focus on the incestuous parent-child relationship by Freud, Jung, and their followers is owing to the fact that so much of the pathology observed by these investigators has had its origins in the damaged parent-child relationship. With the historical deterioration of the sacred bond of marriage, and the loss of connection to the incest mystery, I believe parents have tended to project their soul-mate image (anima or animus)[2] onto their children. For example, when a mother projects her animus onto her son, the son then experiences union with mother as holding the key to his completion. The sexuality which is constellated between mother and son contains all the power and numinosity of the soul-mate attraction. An important consequence of this is that the incest taboo, instead of sanctifying the union between mother and father, functions to repress and contain the forbidden incestuous sexuality. This can be accomplished only by a severe repression which splits sexuality originating in the lower half of the body from the tender, warm, loving, caring feelings originating in the upper half of the body. This splitting between love/sex, upper/lower, spirit/flesh, mind/body, is what I have termed the Incest Wound, which in contrast to Freud's Oedipus complex, is not necessarily a normal stage of development. I believe this type of splitting to be a deeply rooted psychological element in our culture which has gone hand in hand with the deification of the rational mind and a hypertrophied left brain, Apollonian consciousness.

Where Freud views the repression of incestuous sexuality as a normal development process essential for ego formation and the development of culture, I see this repression as a manifestation of a breakdown in marriage, family, and community which has been deeply wounding to our capacity for love and intimacy. For Freud, instincts, including the sexual instinct, are blind drives seeking only to relieve somatic tensions. He equates ego with reason, culture, and sanity; and instincts with uncon-

---

2. The unconscious contrasexual soul image in the psyche, anima for a man, animus for a woman.

trolled passions and animality. How is intimacy possible, I wonder, as long as we mistrust and fear our spontaneous instinctual reactions? The archetypal perspective makes it possible for us to move away from this type of ego-centered psychology because all instincts are viewed as containing a directing intelligence concerned as much with the development of the soul as it is with the life of the body and the survival of the species.

The primary function of the incest prohibition is to stimulate the sexual imagination and to bring the untamed instincts into the service of love and kinship. This is not the same as the *repression* of instincts which seems so necessary in our modern civilization. I believe that when a culture uses repression to control instincts, it has probably lost touch with the meaning of the incest mystery.

Because our culture lacks viable rituals and social forms for regulating the incest libido, the responsibility for preventing incest, for dealing with the whole mystery of incest, has fallen largely onto the individual. Without these protective and integrating rituals, a child is forced to solve by himself a moral conflict involving the deepest mysteries of life. Most of the time this results in a repression of sexuality, but it is not uncommon when there is open sexual provocation by the adult, that the child is unable to repress his sexuality. In these cases the spiritual feelings of warmth and tenderness are repressed. For example, a woman could not remember ever feeling close and loving to her father. Her most poignant memories of him, which she now resented, were primarily related to actual sexual contact and the fantasies which these experiences provoked. In another instance, a man remembers, without the slightest guilt, having had strong sexual desires and fantasies toward his mother; he too could not remember any close or warm moments with her. These examples illustrate that it is not *necessarily* the repression of sexuality, but the love/sex split which is responsible for the incest wound.

Let us explore another common type of experience. When a father projects his soul-mate image or anima onto his daughter, generally owing to a lack of spiritual intimacy with his wife, their connection becomes very strong and basically erotic. Because of the incest fear they can not allow erotic feelings or imagery to enter consciousness. If this repression of sexual imagery and feelings is reasonably successful, there can be a number of consequences:

1. The child becomes unconscious and cut off from her naturally erotic nature. Since she can more easily block out sexual feelings and imagery than control the spontaneous reactions of her body, a split occurs between the upper heart and mind centers and the lower sexual centers of body consciousness;

2. along with the fear and repression of sexuality, the child grad-

ually begins to fear any natural spontaneous expressions of her nature because the "dirty secret" might pop out if she reveals her true self. In other words, the self gets buried along with the forbidden sexuality. With the emerging self blocked, the child develops an identification with a non-threatening self image, which is always false because vital parts of her nature are excluded;

3. because father too must repress his sexuality, he is also fearful of the spontaneous expressions of the self, so he ends up playing the archetypal role of father rather than being himself;

4. with the projection of father's anima onto the daughter, they form an unconscious spiritual marriage which causes another split because the conscious and sexual marriage is with mother. Psychologically, the daughter then falls into the role of the "other woman," and she feels both guilty and superior to mother. On one level she wants to get rid of mother so that she can have father all to herself, but since on another level she needs mother's love, she is thrown into a love/hate ambivalence. But mother too is into a similar love/hate ambivalence because she experiences daughter as the other woman. When the split is severe, this often results in a deep mutual rejection. Many women end up by totally rejecting mother or anything to do with motherhood, and they remain identified with the daughter archetype for the rest of their lives. Because of the repression of the natural self and the fear of revealing it, no one involved in an incestuous triangle is able to be truly herself or himself. Out of her guilt, the daughter may fall into the role of the good and obedient child, or she may feel so betrayed and rejected by mother that she becomes the angry, rebellious child. When her sexuality begins to blossom in puberty, the split becomes even more severe and the relationship to father becomes increasingly fragmented. Often, the desperate need to break away from home is linked to a rejection of the family dynamics and a need to get free of the oppressive soul-splitting incestuous triangle. Instead of experiencing the attraction and harmony between the masculine/feminine opposites, the child experiences these archetypes—sun/moon, yang/yin, heaven/earth, spirit/flesh—as hostile opponents. In psychotherapy, I believe the desperate need to heal this split is often at the core of the so-called transference neurosis.

Depending on the severity of the incest wound, a child may be forced to repress all sexual imagery in order to be sure that none of the guilt-provoking fantasies invade his psyche. Fortunately most children do not have to use such extreme measures, but when they do it results in an over-

175

whelming fear of sexuality and a severe blockage of the sexual instinct. Such children have a tendency to panic at the slightest sign of losing control. More typically children are able to allow non-incestuous sexuality to enter consciousness, but the incest wound still prevents feelings of kinship connection and all the romantic, loving fantasies of spiritual intimacy from entering the psyche along with the sexual imagery. Thus, the incest wound is directly responsible for this common type of internal split between love and sex, between the spiritual and sensual portions of the soul. When the tension between the incest desire and prohibition is obliterated, fragmentation results and the essential internal union between the feminine/masculine opposites is not possible.

I believe the severity of the wound can be measured by the degree of fear one has of losing rational control, even if that fear is not directly related to sexuality. Why is there such horror of losing rational control, of allowing irrational and spontaneous emotions and desires to express themselves without ego censor? Is it because we fear going crazy or committing horrible crimes? What is going on inside when we are caught in this ego trap that makes us so mistrustful of our instincts? I remember a shocking dream I had when I first became aware of the depth of my own incest wound: I go to my office for something. It is late at night, about 11 p.m. As I open the door I suddenly become frightened, sensing some ominous presence in the room. I switch on the light, but see no one. Suddenly, I hear a noise like a whimper coming from behind me. I turn to discover a small, ragged twelve-year-old boy crouching under my desk. I awaken terrified. Later, using the technique of active imagination which Jung suggests, I re-entered the dream in fantasy: I pull the frightened boy out from under my desk and demand to know what he is doing there. At first he refuses to answer, but finally he tells me that he hides under my desk all the time when I see patients. Then turning to me with a lustful grin, he says, "I really dig all those sexy stories your patients tell you." I become furious, call him a sex maniac and threaten to turn him over to the police. Then he breaks down and my heart goes out to him. I take him into my arms. Between sobs he tells me how I had abandoned him when I was twelve because of my own sexual guilt and how I forced him to go underground out of fear of my own lust.

Obviously this little boy was an image of that part of me that I had repressed. One can imagine how fearful I must have been, at the time of this dream, of losing rational control if all of my repressed incestuous sexuality lurked just under the protective front of the physician's desk.

Such examples of the soul-splitting effects of repressed incestuous sexuality are plentiful and relatively easy to grasp once they have been revealed. However, many other expressions of the incest wound are not so obvious. For example, sexual desire may not become fully aroused except in a triangular situation. As soon as the triangle is broken the desire often disappears or diminishes. This may seem contradictory because one would expect that the incest fear would inhibit sexuality in a triangular situation. However, we must not forget that the purpose of the incest taboo is to prevent a child from having sexual union in those relationships where he feels the greatest spiritual intimacy. Thus incest guilt can be avoided as long as one is unaware of experiencing one of the opposites, love or sex. The repressed opposite will, however, continually threaten to re-enter consciousness because of the soul's fundamental need for union. In other words, the *longing for incestuous union, even though it is repressed, is as powerful as is our horror of violating the taboo.* The more we repress the desire the more power it gains over us, so that we are continually fascinated by and falling into incestuous types of involvements. So long as we remain unconscious of the repressed other half, we do not experience the guilt and painful conflict. Innocently we plunge from one relationship to another, emerging each time fragmented and disillusioned.

Another very common manifestation of the incest wound is the experience of loving someone sexually and spiritually in fantasy, but of being cut off or unable to express such feelings in actuality. This situation often occurs because of the fear of consciously embracing the phallic or aggressive aspect of the sexual instinct. The incestuous guilt associated with aggressive sexuality prevents such people from initiating the flow of eros, although they may be very responsive to the initiating action of others. In this way they can remain unconscious of their own aggressive impulses and continue to feel innocent.

As long as the desire for incestuous union remains unconscious it will be activated in every relationship which offers the possibility of soul connection. This has the effect of obstructing the natural, spontaneous flow of love because the incest archetype always demands eternal commitment in a sacred marriage. Simply put, if I feel compelled to make a permanent commitment every time love moves me toward union with another, will this not make me cautious and fearful of loving? One must be free to love or not to love, to feel and express love in the quick of the moment whether or not it lasts forever. The incest wound interferes with this freedom because of the soul's longing for the sacred, eternal union with its mate. This longing for eternal union needs to be experienced as a psychic reality or it will continually interfere with our capacity for intimacy by demanding literal fulfillment whenever one feels love for another.

Apart from love and sex, the incest wound tends to interfere with the experience and spontaneous expression of all the aggressive instincts. Part of this is owing to the fear of losing rational control, but it is also a direct consequence of the guilt-evoking incestuous triangle. A son will fear standing up to his father and revealing his own aggressive potency because of his unconscious incestuous marriage to mother. In the language of Freud's oedipal complex, the guilt and fear of castration arises from the internalized parental authority or superego. The more severe the wound the more the child experiences the inner parent as rejecting of his nature, especially his sexual nature.

Let us not forget that the incest wound refers to the split which occurs in a child's psyche usually as a result of the repression of sexuality in relation to a parental figure. When a parent projects the soul-making ideal onto a child, guilt, fear and repression of sexuality usually occur in both parent and child. As a consequence, the incest archetype splits and the natural, spontaneous, soulful experience of intimacy between parent and child is obstructed. The child will then feel the same incestuous guilt, fear and splitting in any experience in which kinship connection and erotic feelings of intimacy occur simultaneously. The experience of opposition between the parental archetype and erotic intimacy has another important consequence: Since the parental archetypes are responsible for giving the sense of stability, structure and permanency to any relationship, the incest wound tends to cripple the sexual instinct as soon as a relationship begins to feel stable and permanent.

The sacrament of marriage binds the couple to each other and it gives them communal recognition as a social unit committed to mothering and fathering a family of their own. Resistance to marriage is often a fear of falling under the power of the parental archetypes where love becomes a passionless duty and sex becomes a dirty, loveless, masturbatory act. Of course, I am describing the traditional Puritanical split which Freud first observed. Our late-twentieth-century sexual mores have considerably altered this picture so that we are more able to be sexually open and sensually free nowadays without feeling sinful. But the incest wound still makes it difficult for us to open up to the union of love and sex, spirit and body, when the parental archetypes are constellated as they are in marriage. One of the reasons falling in love is such a wonderful experience is that we feel whole and healed and at one with the cosmos. Even the deepest incest wounds are temporarily healed. But as soon as Cupid and Aphrodite move on, the old wounds begin to reappear.

Many couples are able to experience an intimate, vital sexual connection with each other, but their hearts are closed during the sexual act. Before and after intercourse, they may feel tender, caring, protective and spiritually intimate, but it is as if they have to let go of those sentiments in order to get with their sexual passion. Other couples have great difficulty experiencing sexual passion with each other as soon as the love affair is over and the parental archetypes enter, which often occurs on the wedding day. When this happens sexuality may be totally blocked or it tends to be unconnected and masturbatory. This used to be the dominant pattern in our culture, but it seems to be shifting as a result of the cultural acceptance of the joys of sex.

Still, the veins of the incest wound run deep so that marriage relationships tend to become progressively less erotic as couples begin to carry more and more of the parental images for each other. Even in those marriages where the sexual passion is kept alive, I believe this seldom occurs unless the woman has such a strong identification with the Love Goddess and is so cut off from the mother archetype that the mother image is only minimally constellated in the marriage relationship. Such women tend to have disdain for their own mothers and are very rejecting of the mother role for themselves. They also tend to fall heavily into a daughter role with their husbands and with most men. Because of the profound spirit/sex split, these women can often be very open sexually in spite of being into such a father-daughter relationship with their husbands. This is so because the split enables them to be sexually open yet spiritually closed and thus not vulnerable to the threatening father archetype. Consequently their sexuality remains unconscious and therefore unable to enter into the humanizing light of spiritual love.

Since so much of our sexual aggression and passion is contained in our repressed incestuous desires, keeping sexuality alive in a legitimate relationship such as marriage is difficult because only forbidden, illicit erotic imagery can release the repressed instincts. Many couples keep the erotic tensions going by having illicit affairs or by creating jealousy-provoking situations that stimulate the sexual imagination. Some couples use pornographic material to release their sexuality and others can achieve orgasm only when they are able to lose themselves in very specific fantasies. I don't mean to imply that the fascination with images of forbidden sexuality is pathological, but only that the *dependency* on such images for the release of sexuality is a manifestation of the incest wound.

II

Prevalent among older and "primitive" traditions is the notion of two kinds of souls. Plato, for example, describes the soul as consisting of a divine or immortal soul located in the head and a mortal soul located below the neck. According to a Scandinavian school of ethnological research on soul, quoted by Hillman (1979), there is a world-wide experience of two kinds of souls.

> On the one hand, there is the *life-soul* that is multiple, having various associations with body parts and emotions, and so is also called "body-soul," "breath-soul," and "ego-soul." On the other hand, there is a *free-soul*, or *psyche-soul*, also called "image-soul," and "dream-soul." The body-soul and psyche-soul have different natures

and origins, as well as different tasks and spheres of activity. The psyche-soul appears only outside the body and, limited to this form of existence, is out of play in waking, conscious and active states of the person. (pp. 104-105)

It becomes active during sleep, dreams, reverie, visions and shamanistic type of trances.

I have found these ancient notions about the soul invaluable to my understanding of another frequent consequence of the incest wound: the severe loss of connection to the body-soul and the tendency to retreat into the dreamy realm of the disembodied psyche-soul. When the retreat is severe, individuals often have great difficulty adapting to the embodied life of this world. On the other hand, the rejected life-soul also does everything possible to evoke the repressed incestuous sexuality in order to return us to the body. It does this through involving us compulsively in forbidden, illicit sexual fantasies and relationships, and through driving us out of our interior imagistic soul life into a compulsive involvement with external matters.

I believe my own retreat into the disembodied psyche-soul during childhood and adolescence was largely owing to my own incest wound. Even though I was very active physically, I feel I had little connection to my emotional bodily centers. Some time ago, when I was feeling deeply troubled and isolated, I decided to visit the city of my birth where I had lived until the age of ten. As I wandered through the old places I used to frequent, I became aware of having no childhood memories of feeling closely connected to anyone or to any living thing. I was shocked by this realization of how cut off from life I must have been as a child. Although at other times I have been able to recall some childhood memories of closeness with people and nature, I know that I lived mostly in my inner world as a child. I also know that I was very repressed and fearful of my sexuality—for example, not until the age of sixteen do I remember ever touching my penis sensually. At the age of nineteen, I had my first real experience of sexual intimacy. It was incredible. A vital life force filled my body, ensouling it. I felt my body alive with soul and I experienced the body of my partner equally alive with soul, numinous, sacred. I was filled with tenderness, compassion, lust and love. Perhaps for the first time, I felt myself fully entering into the world and at one with it. Of course I fell in love. But more than this, from that time onward my connection to this world and this life became dependent on my having a strong erotic connection to a woman.

If my fear and repression of sexuality in relation to my mother caused me to cut off from an intimate feeling connection to her and from my own warm spontaneous self, is it not understandable that before my natural self could once again enter into an intimate loving connection to a woman, I would need to open up sexually? As long as I feared my embodied soul, as long as the superego or some inner judgmental voice made me fearful of expressing my natural spontaneous self, a barrier to true intimacy was created. In any relationship, when one is able to experience the other person as fully accepting of oneself, the soul temporarily loses its fear of revealing itself and both the repressed erotic nature and the self are released. If this experience leads to sexual intimacy, the erotic flow often becomes intense, and one may feel that nothing is more important in life than maintaining that connection. I believe such erotic dependency is another consequence of the incest wound. However, it is not the intense erotic connection which is so essential to the soul, but the freeing of the repressed natural self, the life-soul, which is made possible by the erotic release. Once the soul is able to overcome its fear of revealing itself, it will lose its dependency on erotic intensity to release it.

As we have seen, the important psychological functions of the incest taboo are as follows:

1. to stimulate the sexual imagination and the formation of the image of Marriage as a Sacred Union, the *hieros gamos*;

2. to humanize and transform sexuality;

3. to make us aware of our incompletion and to stimulate our desire to attain completion, first through union with another, but ultimately through an internal union.

We have been speaking of the soul-splitting effects of the incest wound in terms of mind/body, love/sex, spirit/flesh, upper/lower and so on. Obviously we cannot demonstrate a literal split between mind and body or the upper and lower halves of the body or even the love/sex split. So what we are talking about is an imaginal split. The wound is to the psyche-soul, not the body-soul, although the body will certainly be affected. Since the body-soul is ruled by the pleasure-unpleasure principle, it becomes quickly attached to any material body or object which gives it pleasure. Cut off from the psyche-soul it is incapable of seeing through, of transcending its literal attachments. The objects of the body-soul's desires are also images which are as essential for the nourishment of the psyche-soul as are material objects for the body-soul. As Hillman (1979) puts it, "Every reality of whatever sort is first of all a fantasy image of the psyche" (p. 137). Without the help of the psyche-soul, the body-soul cannot realize that it too is dependent on images for nourishment. The body is not fundamentally attracted to the material substance of the object, but to the images which the object evokes and incarnates. This statement seems obvious when we remember how easily a material object can fascinate and capture us, and how just as easily it can suddenly lose all of its appeal. Yes, we all know this, but the body-soul does not know

181

such things unless it is informed by the psyche-soul, Without this awareness, the body-soul becomes possessive of and possessed by its attachments to material objects. This is what the sin of idolatry is all about: that is, we lose our capacity to see the Great Spirits which enliven the world and therefore we end up worshipping material objects. Materialism, literalism and idolatry go hand in hand.

In our discussion of the incest wound we talked about the importance of forbidden, illicit erotic imagery for the release of repressed incestuous sexuality. Of course, erotic images involving incest are the most forbidden of all. Yet, have I not proposed that a primary function of the incest taboo is to promote the formation and development of such imagery? Perhaps a major consequence of the incest wound is that we become guilty and fearful whenever our consciousness is invaded by any type of "forbidden" thoughts and images, not only erotic ones.

The incest taboo is not meant to make us feel guilty and fearful about our incestuous desires and images. *By inhibiting and protecting us from the desire for literal incest, it allows and encourages complete imaginal freedom.* Perhaps the fear of images and the lack of differentiation between the literal and imaginal in our culture is yet another manifestation of the incest wound. For example, on the level of the body-soul, once the body opens up to sexuality, the instinct can only be fulfilled by literal enactment. On the other hand, the psyche-soul is free to open up to the sexual instinct and to be nourished by the erotic images released even if literal action is not possible or desired. If we fear sexuality in any relationship, eros is obstructed and intimacy is not possible. One of the reasons marriage tends to be so oppressive to the soul is that the fear of violating the vow of sexual fidelity closes us off to intimacy in other relationships. As long as we remain stuck on the body-soul level, it is impossible even to imagine new forms of marriage which will allow both containment and freedom.

We began with the notion that behind the human drive toward coupling are images of the sacred marriage of a divine couple and the soul's sense of incompletion. This search for wholeness through union and permanent coupling with one's soul-mate is, of course, doomed to failure because it is only through the continual process of the internal union of opposites that the soul is able to fulfill its destiny. In this sense, marriage, by binding us to the myth of finding completion through union with another, works in opposition to the soul's need to be free to pursue individuation wherever it leads. These basic human needs to establish permanent bonds and also to be free and unattached are a polarity that can only be resolved when the soul is able to experience being *simultaneously coupled and uncoupled,* which is only possible on the level of the psyche-soul. I have explored this idea in more detail in another paper entitled, "Coupling/Uncoupling."

On the level of the body-soul, bodies really do unite and become one through sexual intimacy. This bodily marriage of souls has been the fundamental bond in the male-female connection and, from the evolutionary perspective, I believe we have not moved much beyond this level. As long as the marriage bond remains on this bodily level, it will always be threatened or broken by extramarital intimacy, with or without sexual involvement. And, as long as our incestuous wounds make us fearful, mistrustful and rejecting of the images arising from our natural body-soul, we will be unable to transcend the literalism of this material plain of existence. Not being able to allow these images to enter consciousness amounts to a rejection of the body-soul. *The incest wound blocks us from the imaginal realization of the body's sensations and experiences.* Every bodily reaction is accompanied by a corresponding image. If the psyche-soul does not have free access to these images, our lives will be dominated by the basic needs of the rejected body-soul in one form or another, i.e., one person may have little or no control over bodily impulses while another may use most of his energy to control them.

What archetypal psychology and all the great religions teach us, in different ways, is that we must free ourselves of our dependency on the material and literal connections to things. The soul becomes free of its bodily bondage, and its bondage to other bodies, when we are able to move to the imaginal, psychic levels of consciousness. Marriage is so oppressive to the free-soul, the psyche-soul, because it cultivates a form of conditional love that binds us possessively to one body. One needs to be able to honor the experience of the Sacred Marriage in sexual union as primarily an imaginal experience of the psyche-soul in order to move beyond this. I see the new form of marriage as one based on an unconditional love that frees the imaginal psyche-soul and deliteralizes the attachments of the body-soul.

REFERENCES

Hillman, J. (1979). *The dream and the underworld.* New York: Harper & Row.
Jung, C. G. (1963). Mysterium coniunctionis. In H. Read, M. Fordham, & G. Adler (Eds.) and R. Hull (Trans.), *The collected works of C. G. Jung* (Vol. 14). Princeton: Princeton University Press/Bollingen Series XX. (Original work published 1955.)
Kroeber, A. L. (1959). Totem and taboo in retrospect. *American Journal of Sociology 65,* 446-51.
Plato. (1952). *Symposium.* New York: Penguin.
Stein, R. (1981). Coupling/uncoupling: Reflections on the evolution of the marriage archetype. *Spring.* Dallas: Spring Publications. (Also published in *Money, food, drink, and fashion and analytic training: The proceedings of the Eighth International Congress for Analytical Psychology,* Berlag Adolk Bonz Gmbll, Fellbach-Oeffingen.)
Stein, R. (1984). *Incest and human love: The betrayal of the soul in psychotherapy.* Dallas: Spring Publications.

Author's Addendum – July 1985

Reflections on the Current Epidemic of Incest, Child Abuse, and Sexual Molestation

Actual child abuse always reflects a lack of connection to and respect for the internal psychic child. As an archetype, the image of the child is associated with a newly developing aspect of the psyche which is still very much contained in nature. As Kerenyi (Kerenyi & Jung, 1949) puts it, being at home in the primeval world is an essential quality of the child archetype (p. 40). The attitude toward the child that we seem to have inherited from Victorian times is that the psyche of a newborn infant is *tabula rasa,* and that the child's development depends entirely on how we educate and shape it. Treating the child as an object to be molded instead of relating to it as an intelligent soul capable of intentionality and choice is, in my view, a psychological root of child abuse. From the studies of abusive parents, we know that the majority have been abused themselves as children and that this abuse has been perpetuated internally by a loveless, critical superego that has no understanding or respect for the inner child.

Freud (1905/1953) destroyed the Victorian image of the child as innocent, pure, virginal, helpless, and asexual in his seminal work, *Three Contributions to the Theory of Sex.* In making us aware of the crucial importance to psychological development of the sexual drive in infancy and childhood, he has paradoxically established that the sexual instinct and probably other basic human instincts contain an intelligence and intentionality that go beyond the mere physical survival of the species. Thus, when a child is blocked or cut off from its sexual instincts as a consequence of the oedipal complex, or what I have termed the incest wound, it loses touch with an instinctual power and intelligence that could protect it from abuse and manipulation.

Depth psychology has shown us that the external and internal worlds reflect each other. If the prevailing epidemic of incest and child abuse is a reflection of our collective attitude toward the child within, then we need to ask oursleves what is behind the compulsive need to abuse and sexually molest the child.

The way I treat my inner child is the way I am going to treat my outer child. Why would I want to abuse my inner child? How do I abuse it? If my child is getting out of hand, I want to stop it and that may result in abuse. For example, my child enjoys just playing and being, it doesn't much like schedules and the pressure which I put on it to work, to write this paper, to do anything that isn't fun. I abuse my inner child primarily by not letting it have its way very often and by putting it down for being so lazy and unproductive. And when it becomes withdrawn and depressed, I do everything possible at first to get it moving, to get it busy doing something worthwhile with its time. The more ego directed and collective are our attitudes and goals, the more trouble are we likely to have with the inner child because the archetypal child contains knowledge about its own developmental needs which is often in opposition to our ego orientation. And, those of us who are not clever enough to manipulate and control the child verbally, often resort to abusive physical measures to keep it in its place.

Paradoxically, an adult's compulsive need for sexual intimacy may initially have arisen out of deep feelings of compassion for the neglected, abused child. What I am suggesting is that the other side of this hate for the troublesome child is a deep love and compassion for this vulnerable, neglected, abandoned, and abused aspect of the soul. The soul's need for union is often expressed in images of sexual intimacy. When an adult suffers from a deep spirit/flesh, mind/body, love/sex split, he or she will often fall under the compulsive power of the sexual drive to literalize these images. Healing does not lie in attempting to overcome these "perverse" desires, but in being able to fully experience the incestuous desires emotionally and imaginally. In this way the sexual drive is gradually transformed and the child (inner and outer) can be loved, honored, and respected as a unique being.

The image of the child as innocent, helpless, unprotected, and lacking a sexual drive seems to be more rooted in the archetype of the innocent divine maiden (Kore) than in the empirical realities of childhood. Persephone, the innocent maiden goddess who is abducted, raped, and carried off to the underworld by Hades represents a charming, seductive quality of the soul which certainly belongs to the child. This innocent, vulnerable, virginal quality of the soul which is so easily violated, and tends even to invite violation from the dark underworld forces, can be seen psychologically as belonging to the soul's need to be penetrated and deepened. This type of penetration from below, which we often experience as rape, needs to be recognized as a psychological process essential to soul-making or it will tend to be lived in literal ways, that is, through identification with the innocent-victim role or through attachment to others upon whom the archetype is projected. Perhaps the current epidemic of child abuse and sexual molestation is also in part owing to the fact that we have projected the Kore archetype onto our children, who then tend to live out this projection for us.

I believe that Alice Miller (1981) in her book, *Prisoners of Childhood,* has described beautifully the child who has identified with this Kore projection and who is, as a consequence, repeatedly violated because it has no access to the ground of its instinctual being. No healthy animal would allow itself to be vulnerable or close to anyone it sensed as abusive; nor would it tolerate for an instant anyone taking advantage of its trust and vulnerability. Why should a healthy child be any less capable of protecting itself? My 3-year-old granddaughter who is as vulnerable and seductive as a playful kitten is also as determined, independent, and powerful as a tiger when she wants her way. Miller's (1984) image of the child as "always innocent" and her rejection of Freud's theories of infantile sexuality as a projection of the Victorian patriarchal attitude toward children, seems to me rather a regression to the pre-Freudian Victorian projection onto the child. I am somewhat shocked that a respected psychoanalyst would reject Freud's drive theory at this particular time and that she would even suggest that this notion has contributed to the perpetuation of child abuse and sexual molestation in our culture.

Is there perhaps a connection between the exploitation and abuse of children in Victorian times and the onset of the industrial age? And is there perhaps a similar connection between the onset of our modern computer age and the epidemic of child abuse? Are we, like our Victorian ancestors, perhaps inflated with our newfound power to understand and manipulate the natural forces of the universe? Are we perhaps identifying with what Jung would call the all-knowing Old Wise Man or Senex archetype? Identification with an archetype always leads to inflation and one-sidedness. Cut off from the renewing vitality of the child archetype, the Senex becomes progressively narrow, arid, and rigid. The greater the internal psychic split between the Senex and Child archetypes, the more desperate is the need of the Senex to unite with those qualities of innocent wonder, openness, vulnerability, and the virginal freshness which the child carries. But the child also needs the stabilizing strength, ancient spiritual wisdom, and depth of the Senex. Thus, Senex and Child are a polarity that function creatively for psychological development only when they form a complementary whole rather than an oppositional split. Such a split is probably a major factor responsible for the compulsive need of so many adults, nowadays, for sexual intimacy with children. As for the child, who, as I suggested, may be living out this projection of the innocent, virginal Kore archetype, not only has it been deprived of its instinctual power to protect itself from such abuse, but it too is in the grips of an archetypal power that is needing to unite with its other half.

My concern about the hysteria being created around this current epidemic of incest and sexual molestation is that it is intensifying the fear of sensuality and sexuality between parent and child instead of inspiring us to find a new, creative relationship to the incest mystery. I have suggested that the primary function of the incest prohibition is to stimulate the sexual imagination and to bring the untamed instincts into the service of love, kinship, and creativity. This means that it is essential to the psychological health and development of the child that it is able to experience an erotic flow and connection to parents and siblings without fear, guilt, or violation.

Let me end these reflections with a few quotes from a superb original paper, *Oedipal Love in the Countertransference,* by Harold Searles (1965) in which he proposes that the mutual experience of romantic and erotic feelings between analyst and analysand is an essential aspect of the resolution of the Oedipus complex in analysis:

> I have found, time after time, that in the course of the work with every one of my patients who has progressed to, or very far towards, a thoroughgoing analytic cure, I have experienced romantic and erotic desires to marry, and fantasies of being married to, the patient. (p. 284)

He indicates that he has experienced the same phenomenon occurring with both sexes (p. 295). Searles offers further evidence to support his concepts through his experience as a husband and parent:

> Towards my daughter, now eight years of age, I have experienced innumerable fantasies and feelings of a romantic-love kind, thoroughly complementary to the romantically adoring, seductive behavior which she has shown toward her father oftentimes ever since she was about two or three years of age. I used at times to feel somewhat worried when she would play the supremely confident coquette with me and I would feel enthralled by her charms; but then I came to the conviction, some time ago, that such moments of relatedness could only be nourishing for her developing personality as well as delightful to me. If a little girl cannot feel herself able to win the heart of her father, her own father who has known her so well and for so long, and who is tied to her by mutual ties, I reasoned, then how can the young woman who comes later have any deep confidence in the power of her womanliness. (p. 296)

REFERENCES

Freud, S. (1953). Three essays on sexuality. In J. Strachey (Ed. and Trans.), *The standard edition of the complete psychological works of Sigmund Freud* (Vol. 7, pp. 125-244). London: Hogarth Press. (Original work published 1905).

Kerenyi, C., & Jung, C. G. (1949). *Essays on a science of mythology.* New York: Pantheon Books.

Miller, A. (1981). *Prisoners of childhood.* New York: Basic Books.

Miller, A. (1984). *Thou shalt not be aware.* New York: Farrar, Strauss, & Giroux.

Searles, H. (1965). Oedipal love in the countertransference. In *Collected papers on schizophrenia and related subjects* (pp. 284-303). New York: International Universities Press. (Original work published 1959).

COMMENT

It is Robert Stein's gift—and contribution to us—to be able to see incest and child abuse from the archetypal perspective. In so doing, he liberates us from the shock, disgust, moral outrage, and consequent righteousness of our mundane ego/superego consciousness.

It is in his Introduction to the Second Edition of *Incest and Human Love* that Robert Stein illuminates the incest-parent-child-sexual-relation issue for me. The archetypal model of incest is brother-sister union. The psychic goal of incest is union with one's *equal* opposite. Seen in this light, the incest epidemic coincides with the dawning of Aquarian consciousness, with the emergence of marriage and of the therapist-patient relationships as partnerships between equally responsible adults. That is what I am living. That is what I am seeing in my work. That is what I am teaching. All the while, I am entertaining endless fantasies of parent-child sex.

It is the soul's "healthy" desire for union/communion with its contrasexual counterpart that leads to a love/sexual union between equally conscious and responsible adults. It is the damaged, wounded ego that can only risk this union with a relatively helpless, dependent, and defenseless child.

My treatment of sexual offenders is based upon my soul's "understanding" that it is equality that the soul seeks and the offender's soul *is* a helpless, dependent, defenseless child. That's why punishment doesn't work, doesn't produce healing. It may work to inhibit behavior and, for many offenders who are irreparably damaged, that is the only realistic goal. Nothing is transformed by punishment. No elevation occurs save possibly the vindication of the victim.

Robert Stein (1984) goes on to say, "I see the development of the Brother-Sister model of psychotherapy as part of a larger evolutionary movement away from the power orientation of patriarchy and matriarchy toward eros-centered models of communal life which promote new levels of intimacy and equality between the sexes" (p. ii). One of these models in which I have immersed myself these past years is the therapeutic community. I see therapeutic community as the emerging structure of all inpatient and residential psychiatric and psychological treatment. Up until the present, most such treatment has been for poor people in public institutions or for very wealthy people in private hospitals. My expectation is that we will see more and more inpatient and eventually outpatient therapeutic-community family-centered psychotherapy for "consenting adults," that is, for people who choose and pay for their own treatment. The core of the therapeutic-community approach is a partnership of equally responsible adults working for the betterment of themselves, each other, and the community as a whole—the place where our children grow up.

REFERENCE

Stein, R. (1984). *Incest and human love, The betrayal of the soul in psychotherapy.* Dallas: Spring Publications.

DONALD LATHROP, M.D.

Arthur L. Rautman

Missed Appointment

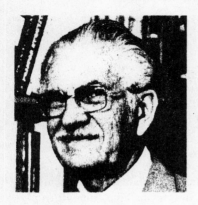

2813 48th Street South
St. Petersburg, Florida 33711

Dr. Rautman has enjoyed clinical work with infants, school children, college students, parents, and adults of all ages; college teaching (including Carleton College and University of Florida); 20 years of clinical work with the psychiatrically disabled (as Chief Clinical Psychologist, U.S. Veterans Administration, Regional Office Mental Hygiene Service, St. Petersburg, Florida); and still, private practice.

Married 49 years, he and Emily have shared the vicissitudes and pleasures of writing for professional journals and of raising their three children, who share their parents' interest in humankind but who delve even deeper into our background: research geology, art history-classical archaeology, and geology-anthropology.

"So this is what it's like. Sit until he gets through with all those guys ahead. Why can't he keep a schedule? I never let my patients sit for hours in the waiting room—except when I couldn't help it, and then I explained and apologized. They never got mad. Oh, well. He probably does the best he can. Seems to be a long line. What a big book! . . . No, it's a computer! Good grief—even here . . .

"Boy, that guy ahead of me seems to be unhappy. Say, he's trying to bribe him to let him in—offering him a pack of stocks and bonds. Let's see if it works. . . . No. . . . It wouldn't do me any good, anyhow . . . I never had any.

"Wonder what it's like in there. Maybe I should have paid more attention in Sunday School on proper procedure. But Dad always said, 'Never mind about all that talk: Just do the best you can and try not to hurt anyone.'

"I thought that's what I did. . . . At least I did the best I could. Once, when I got my degree, he said he was almost proud of me. But he added, 'Don't exploit others just because now you think you are smart enough that you could.'

"I wish I could ask him what to do next. He must have gone through all this same routine some 50 years ago . . . I hope he made it."

"You are next, Sir."

"Oh, O.K. Dad, here I go. Help me if you can. If not, keep me from making an ass of myself."

"Welcome back home, Sir."

"Oh, yes. Thank you. I don't quite know . . . don't quite see what is expected of me . . ."

"No sweat. Just have a seat and make yourself comfortable while I go over some of this stuff. Standard procedure, you know."

"So I've been told."

"Oh, here you are. Quite a long list, I see."

"Oh, I guess . . ."

"Don't worry. I'll go over some of these items with you if I don't understand."

"I'll be glad to explain . . ."

Oh, no. It's all here. We can't add or subtract. My job is to score each item and come up with a total. Something like your Graduate Record exam."

"We scored that on a machine."

"Yes, I know. But we have to assign human values to each item; no machine can do that. After that we stick it into a machine, too. But only for the tabulation. We don't trust value judgments to a machine."

"Oh."

"Let's see here. You've got quite a list of. . . . Did you want me to go over them with you?"

"No, no. I try to forget those . . ."

"Probably not necessary. Petty things . . . kid stuff . . . Hmmm . . . What about this one?"

"Let me see. . . . Oh, yes, I remember. It bothered me for years, but I never did anything about it. What's that checkmark behind it? What does that mean?"

"Oh, we have a system somewhat like your double-entry bookkeeping: We record and score the temptation; and if you carry it out, we record it here on the minus-Brownie-point side. If you do not act on it, we give you a positive score in this column. The value of the points is assigned quite arbitrarily. Negative if you act on it—positive if you don't."

"Is this something new? I was told in Sunday School that you recorded only acts, not . . ."

"No, we've had it for years; we just don't advertise it. Our machine has total recall: It records all acts, thoughts—conscious and unconscious. We know what you people are like. We recognize that you carry motives that had value sometime in your background but that are no longer suitable. It's not what you carry from primitive times, but what you *select*. . . . Say, you've got quite a list of things here. What did you do for a living, anyhow?"

"I was a clinical psychologist. I tried to . . ."

"Oh, yes. I see here. I had overlooked it. Say, you must often have been tempted to interfere in the lives of your patients."

"But I tried to keep . . ."

"Yes, I see. You know, your patron saint, Freud, almost out-guessed our recording system. He saw that you people carried all the past on your backs and needed to recognize both the good and the bad—and to select. I guess he felt that if you were unaware of your own bad side, you could be overwhelmed at times—by surprises."

"I tried . . ."

"Of course, you did. . . . Here's a note about a guy who was trapped for years on an island at war, and couldn't get off. He says here that you promised to help him build a boat, but never did."

"I tried to do . . ."

"Excuse me. I'll give it a flashback."

"Oh, yes. Thanks . . ."

"Well, he said he has been off the island for years now. But he also admits that you never did help him build that boat."

"How did he get off the island, then?"

"He says you carried him in your arms."

"Oh."

"I guess that deserves a double bonus."

"Gee, thanks . . ."

"I see another item I can't quite understand: It's about a young girl—a patient of yours. She wasn't quite sure who or what she was—or who you were. Didn't know what she was to you, or you to her. Guess I'll give it a look-see . . ."

"O.K. Thanks."

"I guess she still thinks you are one of the best persons she ever knew. Says you taught her the difference between loving and being in love."

"Oh."

"Say, she's quite a girl now. I guess that's worth several extra points."

"I was quite concerned . . ."

"Of course. Say, you must have been an imaginative guy. . . . You sure didn't miss many temptations."

"But I tried to help others—not hurt them."

"So I see. Most of your kind think they are being good because they never had an opportunity to be bad. They don't do anything wrong because they are too dull to recognize a temptation—or an opportunity to do good, either, for that matter."

"Uhhhhh . . ."

"Say, you must have had a lot of fun. You seem to have loved so many things—but left them free. By the way, did that mourning dove on that drain-pipe shelf ever get her babies hatched?"

"Eh? Oh, yes."

"Good. And here's another whole list. . . . What's this silly note about a teacup?"

"I only carried it around in my head for years . . ."

"Yes, I see that. She says she has been happy to keep you company."

"Ummm . . ."

"And here are two yellow butterflies that send you greetings and welcome. And here's a note from a rabbit: He says you shot him, but he forgives you. He says your tears on the snow enabled him to live forever in your memory. . . . Says he is quite happy to see you again."

"I . . ."

"Well, welcome back home. You'll find all your friends here waiting for you. They are all in your head, you know. Have a good time."

"Can I come in now?"

"Oh, sure. With you it was just a formality. We wanted you to understand our system of scoring Brownie points."

"Gee, thanks."

*　　*　　*

"Ye gods, What a dream! . . . I do hope my next patient will be on time this afternoon—or I might have another dream. They could change their minds, you know."